Reeder and Felson's

n

Neuroradiology

Compliments of...

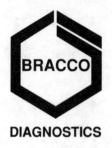

DIAGNOSTICS

REEDER AND FELSON'S

GAMUTS IN NEURO-RADIOLOGY

COMPREHENSIVE LISTS OF
ROENTGEN AND MRI DIFFERENTIAL DIAGNOSIS

MAURICE M. REEDER
WILLIAM G. BRADLEY, JR.

Springer-Verlag

New York Berlin Heidelberg London Paris
Tokyo Hong Kong Barcelona Budapest

Maurice M. Reeder, M.D., F.A.C.R.
Professor and Chairman, Section of Radiology, John A. Burns
    School of Medicine, University of Hawaii at Manoa,
    Honolulu, HI, USA;
Colonel, Medical Corps, United States Army, Retired;
Formerly Chief, Department of Radiology, Walter Reed Army
    Medical Center;
Formerly Radiology Consultant to the Surgeon General, United
    States Army;
Formerly Associate Radiologist, Registry of Radiologic
    Pathology, Armed Forces Institute of Pathology, Washington,
    DC, USA;
Founding Member, International Skeletal Society

William G. Bradley, Jr., M.D., Ph.D., F.A.C.R.
Director, MRI and Radiology Research, Long Beach Memorial
    Medical Center, Long Beach, CA, USA
Professor-in-Residence, Department of Radiological Sciences,
    University of California, Irvine, Orange, CA, USA

Catalog records for this book are available from the U.S. Library of Congress.

Printed on acid-free paper.

Production managed by Karen Phillips; manufacturing supervised by
    Jacqui Ashri.
Photocomposed copy prepared from the authors' WordPerfect file using
    Ventura Publisher.
Printed and bound by Edwards Brothers, Inc., Ann Arbor, MI.
Printed in the United States of America.

9 8 7 6 5 4 3

ISBN 0-387-94034-0 Springer-Verlag New York Berlin Heidelberg
ISBN 3-540-94034-0 Springer-Verlag Berlin Heidelberg New York

Dedication

This book is dedicated to Colonel William LeRoy Thompson, Medical Corps, U.S. Army (1891-1975)

Colonel Thompson, legendary teacher of morphology in radiology and originator of the Gamut concept, received his M.D. degree from the University of Pennsylvania in 1917, and began his long and illustrious career in the U.S. Army Medical Corps that same year. He had various assignments in general medicine and administration and later became one of the early Army radiologists.

It was during his last year before retirement from the Army (1951), however, that he began his most important work, his major contribution to medicine: the organization of the Registry of Radiologic Pathology at the Armed Forces Institute of Pathology. After retirement, he offered his services, without remuneration, to continue as full-time Registrar and Chief of Radiologic Pathology.

In the ensuing 16 years, Colonel Thompson worked laboriously in accessioning new material and collating the material already in the files of the Institute. He was sustained in this labor by hours of daily contact with his "students." It was here, in seminars at the viewbox, that Colonel Thompson drew upon a lifetime of accumulated knowledge and experience to educate residents, fellows, and practicing physicians from all over the world who came to study under his guidance. In this role, Colonel Thompson was the catalyst, igniting in his students a love of learning and an understanding of the vital role that pathology plays in the discipline of radiology. He was primarily a morphologist, and accepted as such by his colleagues and peers at the AFIP.

Colonel Thompson's down-to-earth nature, his éclat in interpersonal relationships, his obvious deep regard for his students as well as medicine, and his abundant and abiding warmth as a human being have made him truly beloved by all who came to know him.

A Tribute to Ben Felson

He was certainly the greatest radiologist of his time, and perhaps of all time. He was one of the great men of this century. He was also my very close and dear friend and colleague. He was like a second father to me and his loss to me is monumental, as is his loss to all whose lives he touched in such a profound and positive manner. He lived the fullest life of anyone I ever knew. He was the quintessential student and teacher, the consummate traveler, and the most compassionate, loving, and lovable human most of us have ever known.

He was that rare combination of Will Rogers and William Osler, and wherever he went, from Cincinnati to Colombia to China, he made a lasting impact and lifelong friends. More than anyone else, he enhanced the reputation and knowledge of the fledgling speciality of Radiology through his inquisitiveness and his gift for communication with both the written and spoken word. He nurtured the careers of countless students, residents, and doctors around the world. He will live forever in the hearts and minds of all who knew and loved him.

Godspeed Ben, and continue to smile down on us from above as you did so often during your all-too-brief stay with us on earth.

Maurice Reeder, M.D.

Foreword to *Gamuts in Radiology,* Third Edition

by Elias G. Theros, M.D.
I. Meschan Distinguished Professor of Radiology,
Wake Forest University Medical Center,
Winston-Salem, North Carolina, USA

Amongst the present generation of radiologists, beguiled by the glamour and excitement of the new high tech imaging and interventional modalities, too few have developed a strong sense of differential diagnosis based on radiologic pattern recognition and its correlation with clinical and laboratory findings. There is no question about the incredible contribution by the new modalities to our diagnostic armamentarium, but in the evolution of modern-day radiologic practice, the cognitive element has been neglected and our abilities as diagnosticians have suffered.

The advent of the third edition of Reeder and Felson's *Gamuts in Radiology* is timely and welcome. As always, use of the gamut lists will help evoke differential thinking, and this has been enhanced by the addition of numerous new gamuts as well as by the updating of over three-fourths of the previously existing gamuts. Interestingly, about 110 of the new gamuts are MRI Gamuts developed by Dr. William Bradley whose enormous experience in clinical MRI and neuroradiology has prepared him to think differentially about look-alike patterns and/or locations of lesions displayed by this modality. This is an important step forward in the use of this remarkable new diagnostic tool.

Drs. Reeder and Felson in preparing these gamuts have made a major contribution to diagnosis in radiology. This they were able to do because of the depth of their own experience and their powers of observation. Those of us who have worked closely with them know that they are radiologists of consummate skills, both in the teaching and practice settings. They are master teachers to whom we all owe much. It is radiology's great fortune that Dr. Reeder has persisted, after Dr. Felson's untimely death, in laboring long hours in gamut researching and updating. He is providing his professional colleagues with an ever improving powerful diagnostic tool. We are all in his debt.

Table of Contents

B

C

H

S

M

Preface

The word *gamut* is defined as the whole range of anything. As used in this book, it indicates a complete list of causes of a particular roentgen finding or pattern.

This book, which consists of material excerpted and reorganized from *Reeder and Felson's Gamuts in Radiology, Third Edition,* was created specifically for neuroradiologists, neurosurgeons, and neurologists. If used correctly, it will become an indispensable aid to pattern recognition and differential diagnosis when interpreting radiographs in the clinical setting.

Most radiologists use the "Gamut approach" without calling it that. You see an enlarged sella turcica and immediately search your memory bank for causes. You recall perhaps six causes, then eliminate two because of rarity or incompatible roentgen pattern. Then, with the clinical information at your elbow, you weed out two more that don't fit the clinical setting, leaving you with perhaps one or two likely diagnoses.

This process is the basis of the triangulation approach to radiologic diagnosis espoused by the originator of the gamut concept, Colonel William LeRoy Thompson. He taught that roentgen diagnosis begins with accurately interpreting all the nuances and data inherent in the radiograph, then using that information to derive a particular pattern. The second side of the triangle involves reference to a well-constructed list of differential diagnosis, which includes not only the common causes, responsible for over 80 percent of the entities, but also the uncommon causes, which are frequently overlooked. The triangle is then completed by reference to the pertinent clinical and laboratory data, age, sex, and other important information concerning the patient.

The purpose of this book is to provide you with complete and accurate lists of differential diagnosis. It is an unobtrusive consultant, quickly available whenever you interpret

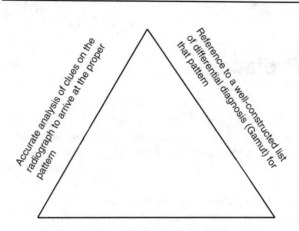

Correlation of radiographic findings
and Gamut with patients clinical
and lab findings to arrive at the
most likely diagnosis

films or prepare a presentation. In each patient, the possibilities are narrowed down to those that fit the roentgen signs and the clinical and laboratory findings. Of course, all the pertinent data on the film must be analyzed to find the appropriate roentgen sign or pattern. Study well — to identify a pattern incorrectly will land you in the wrong gamut, which could be a disaster!

Many individual gamuts that first appeared in *Gamuts in Radiology* can also be found reproduced (credited or otherwise) in a variety of publications. Many excellent texts have been published that emphasize the gamut or differential diagnosis approach, including those by Drs. Eisenberg, Swischuk, Greenfield, Poznanski, Taybi and Lachman, and Burgener and Kormano. However, residents and practitioners who use abbreviated lists from other, more watered-down, sources are deprived of the true worth of gamuts, which is to provide a comprehensive listing of the multiple causes, both common and uncommon, for a particular pattern. The point is to jog your memory to recall *all* the various possibilities for any given finding.

We are the first to admit that the amount of information and knowledge required to analyze with unerring accuracy and completeness all of the patterns which can present to the radiologist is beyond the comprehension of any two (or perhaps twenty) individuals. Nevertheless, our combined experience of over 100 years' practice in major medical centers in the United States (including that of Ben Felson, the esteemed co-author of the complete *Gamuts in Radiology* text), as well as numerous visiting professorships throughout virtually the entire world, have given us sufficient perspective to at least attempt such a prodigious endeavor. Along the way we have been greatly aided by our close association with many outstanding radiologists who broadened our horizons and added invaluable insights in their own specialty areas.

While the individual gamuts are extensively referenced, you will note that the majority of current references refer to textbooks rather than journal articles. This is because today's general and subspecialty textbooks are much more likely to refer to the multiple causes for a given pattern than individual articles, which are usually focused on specific entities or procedures. Furthermore, exhaustive lists of references would increase the book's size enormously and undermine its primary goal, which is to provide a quick, efficient reference.

You may question whether a specific listed entity can give rise to a given pattern, or whether it is a common or uncommon member of that gamut. Although there may be some errors among the many thousands of entries, virtually all listed causes have appeared in the literature or have been seen by the authors or our colleagues. Obviously, what is common in one part of the world may be rare or unknown elsewhere. For example, cysticercosis is perhaps the most common cause of a mass in the brain in Mexico, but it is relatively rare in the northern United States. Multiple sclerosis, on the other hand, is relatively common in the northern latitudes of North America and Europe, but is uncommon in the tropics. Thus, while the list of causes for a specific pattern may be quite complete within each gamut, the relative prevalence of those causes can vary widely geographically.

The legendary Colonel Thompson is well remembered by his former students and disciples for his insistence on the triangulation approach to radiographic interpretation. This clinically oriented physician taught an entire generation of radiology residents and fellows the nuances of interpretation and differential diagnosis of various roentgen patterns. In today's clinical setting, where the proliferation of new technologies is colliding with ever increasing pressures to contain costs and optimize the use of diagnostic tests (as Dr. Theros has so eloquently stated in his foreword), it is more important than ever that young radiologists and clinicians learn and apply these principles, which are summarized in these remarks by the Colonel:

"The radiograph is to the radiologist what the gross specimen is to the pathologist. It is a window on the disease, mirroring the many changes occurring within the patient during the course of an illness."

"The clues to the pattern (and often the diagnosis itself) are almost always on the film if you are observant enough and smart enough to pay attention to all the data inherent in the radiograph."

"Remember that the radiograph is only one-tenth of a second in the history of a disease process. You must always think back to what the findings looked like a day or a week or a year ago (preferably with the help of old films if available, but using intuition or deductive reasoning in their absence) and think ahead to what the findings are likely to be tomorrow or next week."

"A good radiologist must be a good anatomist and morphologist and have a clear understanding of the correlation between what is seen on the radiograph and the underlying gross and microscopic pathology."

Finally, we would like to add a few of our own thoughts that we have passed on to residents over the years.

"The radiograph is only one piece of the diagnostic puzzle. It must be evaluated in light of what you know about the patient. The radiologist cannot function as an isolated island unto himself. He or she needs a knowledge of differential diagnosis together with clinical information and interaction with the patient's physician to arrive at the proper solution."

"The radiograph is like a single page in a mystery novel. To find out 'whodunit' you usually need more detailed information than is available at a single glance."

"Remember that what comes out of the automatic processor so often is not a diagnosis but rather a diagnostic challenge, a pattern for which there may be four or forty possible causes. It is up to us, as the physician's consultant, to interpret this pattern correctly using the triangulation approach."

"With newer modalities such as MRI, it is becoming increasingly important to be conversant with the science behind the images (eg, T1 and T2 changes)."

In sum, the ideal radiologist should combine exceptional visual acuity with the intuition of a good detective, the solid background of a scientist, and the knowledge of odds of a smart card player. It is these qualities and attention to detail that set him or her apart from others who merely "look at" films.

MMR
WGB

Acknowledgments

In creating a project of this magnitude, the authors will inevitably borrow freely from many sources. Specific citations follow most gamuts, and a list of more general references appears at the end of this volume. For those instances where debts are not acknowledged, the reader should understand that lost notes and jaded memories, not ingratitude, are to blame.

The published works of the following outstanding radiologists resulted in valuable additions to many of the gamuts found in this book: Drs. Scott W. Atlas, Michael Brant-Zawadzki, Francis A. Burgener, G. H. DuBoulay, Ronald L. Eisenberg, A. N. Hasso, V. Houghton, S. H. Lee, Thomas H. Newton, G. M. Shoukimas, Peter M. Som, Leonard E. Swischuk, Hooshang Taybi, Louis Teresi, June Unger, G. E. Valvasorri, and, of course, Benjamin Felson, the renowned co-author of the two previous editions of the complete *Gamuts in Radiology* text. We want to especially thank Dr. Elias G. (Lee) Theros for his insightful foreword to this text.

The production and distribution of this book would not have been possible without the unwavering faith and guidance of the Editorial and Book Production staffs of Springer-Verlag New York, who kept the project on track to assure the timely publication of a highly refined end product. Finally, this text would not be possible in its present format without the meticulous and dedicated typing and word processing skills provided by Mrs. Karen Kurihara of Honolulu and Kaye Finley of Long Beach.

An Appreciation

To my wife, Barbara, whose patience, love, and perseverance made possible the timely publication of this present work, and to the entire Reeder family, and to those colleagues, mentors, and friends, past and present, who have so indelibly defined my own career:

> *William LeRoy Thompson*
> *Benjamin Felson*
> *Elias G. Theros*
> *Philip E. S. Palmer*
> *Harold G. Jacobson*

MMR

To my wife, Rosalind B. Dietrich, M.D., and my children, David, Kristin, India, and Felicity, for giving me the time to complete the MRI gamuts.

WGB

How To Use This Book

1. SECTIONS

This book is organized in five sections. Each section is denoted by an alphabetical letter. Thus, under S you will find all the gamuts that deal with the vertebral column or spine.

2. TABLE OF CONTENTS

This book has an extensive index. In addition, each section has its own table of contents, the pages of which have been black-edged for quick recognition. You can identify the appropriate table of contents by referring to page ix or by counting down the black index marks along the free edge of the closed book.

It will pay you to take a few minutes to look over the subheadings in the table of contents of each section. Gamuts are grouped in what we consider a logical manner. However, our logic may not be your logic; if you don't find a gamut where you think it belongs, scan the entire table of contents of that section or refer to the index before assuming that it is absent.

3. SUBGAMUTS

A subgamut amplifies some part of the gamut to which it belongs. Be sure to refer to it after you have finished with the parent gamut.

4. INCIDENCE

In most of the gamuts, the entities are subdivided into two groups, *Common* and *Uncommon*. These refer to the relative, rather than absolute, incidence of the disease. Although an enlarged brain stem (Gamut B-24) is an uncommon roentgen finding, if you do see one, the diagnosis will generally prove to be glioma, hemorrhage, or metastasis as listed under *Common*. However, there are at least ten other *Uncommon* entities that must be considered in the differential diagnosis.

The prevalence of many disorders varies both geographically and from one type of institution to another. Spinal tuberculosis is a common bone disease in much of the world, but it is only occasionally seen in the U.S. Syringomyelia is much more commonly seen at Walter Reed Army Hospital than it is in a county hospital. To avoid such discrepancies, we have based our incidence estimates on our experience at Theoretical General Hospital, Midland, U.S.A.

Admittedly, some of the gamuts deal with seldom seen roentgen signs, but it is in just this type of situation that a gamut is most welcome. It substitutes someone else's experience for your own lack of it.

5. ALPHABETICAL LISTING

The entries in each gamut have been alphabetized for your convenience. Since the entry may not be listed in the form that first comes to your mind, be sure to scan the entire gamut before assuming that a condition is not included. Abbreviations are listed on page 327.

6. SUPPLEMENTARY GAMUTS

Most of the gamuts refer to a roentgen sign, pattern, or complex. However, interspersed throughout the book are classifications, anatomic and physiologic gamuts, and other information useful to the radiologist and clinician. Typical examples are Gamuts B-6A (Incidence of Brain Tumors) and M-14A (Causes of Cerebral Emboli).

7. TERMINOLOGY

We have usually selected the most widely used terms for each disease, often furnishing a synonym or eponym as well.

The term *generalized* indicates more or less diffuse involvement (eg, thalassemia of the skeleton); *widespread* means extensive but spotty involvement (eg, Paget's disease of the skeleton); *multiple* means more than one lesion but less than widespread (eg, metastatic lesions).

In order to shorten the gamut lists, similar or related conditions are combined, often separated by a comma or semicolon (eg, syringomyelia; hydromyelia). Inclusive group designations, such as lymphoma or neurogenic neoplasms, are often utilized. In these instances you will find the subscript $_g$, which tells you to look in the Glossary (page 329) if you want to know all the entities in that group. Example: Neuromuscular disorders$_g$. If one member of a group is a more likely cause of a particular roentgen finding, it is specifically listed. To illustrate: neuromuscular disorders$_g$ (esp. poliomyelitis).

8. BRACKETS

Brackets are used to indicate a condition that does not actually cause the gamuted roentgen finding, but can produce roentgen changes that simulate it. In Gamut M-25 (Pineal Region Tumor), benign cystic pineal gland, which is not a cause, but a mimic, is bracketed.

9. SYNDROMES

S. stands for Syndrome. We must apologize for the great number of congenital syndromes we have included. Since the information is available, we could hardly ignore it. Lump them together? The pediatric roentgenologists had just split them apart. We had a huge tiger by the tail, an animal with variegated stripes and swollen gamuts. Seckel's bird-headed dwarfism, Cockayne, and Prader-Willi syndromes, indeed! They should have their own Gamut Book. We can only advise those of you who seldom see dwarfs and other little people to ignore these entries. For those who are interested, it will be useful to consult Taybi and Lachman's syndrome book for definitions of these congenital disorders.

10. REFERENCES

References are used to cite only articles, books, and other contributions that have provided a number of the disease entities listed in a gamut. To document each entity would be an impossible task. A listing of general references appears in the back of the book.

11. ALTERATIONS

We are fully aware that there are omissions on the Gamut lists. Very rare entities or syndromes or single case reports

have been deliberately omitted. There are also some incon-
sistencies in terminology, coverage, and unity. There may
even be occasional factual inaccuracies. We hope these
flaws are neither too frequent nor too annoying.

Please correct errors if you encounter them; delete entities that you feel do not belong on a gamut; insert additional
disorders and add new gamuts as you discover them in the
literature or in your practice; create some gamuts yourself.
Send us your changes, with documentation, so that they can
be incorporated in future editions.

Roentgen Based Gamuts

B

Brain
(See Section "M" for MRI of the Brain)

VARIOUS PATTERNS SEEN ON CT OR MRI (OTHER THAN MASSES)
(See Section "M" for MRI Evaluation of Brain Lesions)

B

B

Gamut B-1

SOLITARY INTRACRANIAL CALCIFICATION
(See Gamuts B-2 to B-5)

PHYSIOLOGIC
1. Arachnoid granulation, pacchionian body
2. Basal ganglia, dentate nucleus
*3. Choroid plexus
*4. Dura (eg, falx, tentorium, superior sagittal sinus)
*5. Habenular commissure
6. Hypophysis
*7. Interclinoid ligament (diaphragma sellae)
*8. Petroclinoid ligament
*9. Pineal
10. Pituitary "stone"

INFECTION
1. Encephalitis, meningitis, brain abscess (healed)
2. Fungus disease$_g$ (esp. cryptococcosis)
3. Granuloma, congenital cerebral
4. Parasitic cyst (eg, cysticercus, hydatid, paragonimus)
5. Syphilitic gumma
*6. Tuberculosis (eg, tuberculoma, healed meningitis)

NEOPLASM
*1. Chordoma
2. Choroid plexus papilloma
*3. Craniopharyngioma
4. Dermoid, teratoma
5. Ependymoma
6. Epidermoid
*7. Glioma (eg, low-grade astrocytoma, oligodendroglioma)
8. Hamartoma
9. Hemangioma
10. Lipoma of corpus callosum

11. Meningioma
12. Metastatic neoplasm (eg, from osteosarcoma, mucinous adenocarcinoma of colon)
13. Neurinoma
*14. [Osteoma, chondroma, osteochondroma, osteosarcoma, chondrosarcoma]
15. Pinealoma
16. Pituitary adenoma (esp. chromophobe)

VASCULAR

1. Aneurysm (incl. vein of Galen)
*2. Arteriosclerosis (esp. carotid siphon)
*3. Hemangioma, AV malformation, Sturge-Weber S.

MISCELLANEOUS

*1. [Artifact; foreign body; calcified sebaceous cyst]
 2. Hematoma, chronic (eg, intracerebral, subdural, epidural)
 3. [Iatrogenic (eg, contrast medium injection into an abscess or cyst)]
*4. Idiopathic
 5. Infarct, cerebral
 6. Porencephalic cyst
 7. Radiation necrosis
 8. Scarring; gliosis
 9. Tuberous sclerosis

*Common.

References:

1. DuBoulay GH: Principles of X-ray Diagnosis of the Skull (ed 2) London: Butterworths, 1980, pp 244-283
2. Newton TH, Potts DG: Radiology of the Skull and Brain. St. Louis: C.V. Mosby, 1971, vol 1, book 2, pp 823-873
3. Swischuk LE: Differential Diagnosis in Pediatric Radiology. Baltimore: Williams & Wilkins, 1984, pp 372-376
4. Teplick JG, Haskin ME: Roentgenologic Diagnosis. (ed 3) Philadelphia: W.B. Saunders, 1976, vol 2

Gamut B-2

MULTIPLE INTRACRANIAL CALCIFICATIONS
(See Gamuts B-1, B-4)

COMMON

1. Atherosclerosis
2. Idiopathic
3. Physiologic (eg, dura, falx, tentorium, petroclinoid ligament, diaphragma sellae, choroid plexi, pineal, habenula)

UNCOMMON

1. AV malformation; aneurysms; hemangiomas; Sturge-Weber S.; von Hippel-Lindau disease
2. Basal cell nevus S. (falx, tentorium)
3. Basal ganglia (eg, hypoparathyroidism; pseudo-hypoparathyroidism; Fahr disease) (See B-4)
4. Brain abscesses (healed)
5. Calcinosis, metastatic
6. Carbon monoxide intoxication
7. Cockayne S.
8. Cytomegalic inclusion disease
9. Encephalitis (eg, measles, rubella, chickenpox, neo-natal herpes simplex, polio)
10. Folic acid deficiency
11. Fungus disease$_g$ with basal arachnoiditis (eg, cryptococcosis, coccidiomycosis)
12. Hematomas, old (eg, intracerebral, subdural)
13. Homocystinuria
14. Hyperparathyroidism, primary or secondary-renal failure (vascular calcifications)
15. Hypervitaminosis D (dura, pineal)
16. [Iatrogenic (eg, Pantopaque or other contrast medium residual)]
17. Idiopathic hypercalcemia (Williams S.) (falx, tentorium)
18. Lead poisoning

19. Leukemia (treated)
20. Lipoid proteinosis (hyalinosis cutis)
21. Lissencephaly (congenital agyria)
22. Listeriosis
23. Methotrexate therapy
24. Needle-tracks following ventriculography
25. Neoplasms, multiple (eg, meningiomas, gliomas, metastases)
26. Neurofibromatosis (choroid plexi)
27. Parasitic disease (eg, cysticercosis, paragonimiasis, hydatid disease)
28. Pseudoxanthoma elasticum
29. [Scalp (eg, sebaceous cysts, cysticercosis, foreign bodies, EEG paste)]
30. Scarring; gliosis (eg, postradiation therapy; old trauma)
31. Toxoplasmosis
32. Tuberculomas; tuberculous meningitis (treated)
33. Tuberous sclerosis
34. Wilson's disease

References:

1. Babbitt DP, Tang T, Dobbs J, et al: Idiopathic familial cerebrovascular ferrocalcinosis (Fahr's disease) and review of differential diagnosis of intracranial calcification in children. AJR 1969;105:352-358
2. Bentson JR, Wilson GH, Helmer E, et al: Computed tomography in intracranial cysticercosis. J Comput Assist Tomogr 1977;4:464-471
3. DuBoulay GH: Principles of X-ray Diagnosis of the Skull. (ed 2) London: Butterworths, 1980, pp 244-283
4. Kumpe DA, Rao CV, Garcia JH, et al: Intracranial neurosarcoidosis. J Comput Assist Tomogr 1979;3:324-330
5. Legré J, Massad A: Radiological study of intracranial calcifications. Radiology 1958;70:760 (abstract)
6. Newton TH, Potts DG: Radiology of the Skull and Brain. St. Louis: C.V. Mosby, 1971, vol 1, book 2, pp 823-873
7. Reyes PF, et al: Intracranial calcification in adults with chronic lead exposure. AJR 1986;146:267-270
8. Schubiger O, Valavanis A, Hayek J: Computed tomography in cerebral aneurysms with special emphasis on giant intracranial aneurysms. J Comput Assist Tomogr 1980;1:24-32
9. Swischuk LE: Differential Diagnosis in Pediatric Radiology. Baltimore: Williams & Wilkins, 1984, pp 372-376

10. Taybi H, Lachman RS: Radiology of Syndromes, Metabolic Disorders, and Skeletal Dysplasias. (ed 3) Chicago: Year Book Medical Publ, 1990, p 860
11. Teplick JG, Haskin ME: Roentgenologic Diagnosis. (ed 3) Philadelphia: W.B. Saunders, 1976

Gamut B-3

SELLAR OR PARASELLAR CALCIFICATION

COMMON

1. Aneurysm of a cerebral artery (eg, internal carotid, circle of Willis, basilar artery)
2. Atherosclerosis of internal carotid artery
3. Craniopharyngioma
4. Normal (petroclinoid or interclinoid ligament-diaphragma sellae)

UNCOMMON

1. AV malformation
2. Cholesteatoma
3. Chordoma
4. Ectopic pinealoma, teratoma
5. Hyperparathyroidism (vascular calcification)
6. Meningioma
7. Optic chiasm glioma
8. [Osteochondroma, chondroma, osteoma]
9. Pituitary adenoma (esp. chromophobe)
10. Pituitary "stone" in otherwise normal pituitary gland
11. Tuberculous meningitis, healed

Reference:
1. DuBoulay GH: Principles of X-ray Diagnosis of the Skull. (ed 2) London: Butterworths, 1980

Gamut B-4

BASAL GANGLIA CALCIFICATION

COMMON

1. Hypoparathyroidism, pseudohypoparathyroidism
2. Idiopathic; normal variant

UNCOMMON

1. Amaurotic idiocy
2. Birth anoxia
3. Carbon monoxide intoxication
4. Cockayne S.
5. Cytomegalic inclusion disease
6. Encephalitis (eg, rubella, measles, chickenpox)
7. Fahr disease (ferrocalcinosis)
8. Familial idiopathic symmetrical basal ganglia calcification
9. Hemorrhage
10. Hyperparathyroidism
11. Hypothyroidism
12. Idiopathic lenticulodentate calcification (Hastings-James S.)
13. Lead encephalopathy
14. Lipoid proteinosis (hyalinosis cutis)
15. Oculo-dento-osseous dysplasia
16. Parasitic disease (eg, toxoplasmosis, cysticercosis)
17. Parkinsonism
18. Pseudopseudohypoparathyroidism
19. Radiation therapy
20. Trisomy 21 S. (Down S.)
21. Tuberous sclerosis
22. Vascular disease (eg, atherosclerosis)

References:

1. Bennett JC, Maffly RH, Steinbach HL: The significance of bilateral basal ganglia calcification. Radiology 1959;72: 368-378
2. Cohen CR, Duchesneau PM, Weinstein MA: Calcification of the basal ganglia as visualized by computed tomography. Radiology 1980;134:97-99

3. Harwood-Nash DCF, Reilly BJ: Calcification of the basal ganglia following radiation therapy. AJR 108:392-395
4. Newton TH, Potts DG: Radiology of the Skull and Brain. St. Louis: C.V. Mosby, 1971, vol 1, book 2, p 835
5. Numaguchi Y, Hoffman JC Jr, Sones PJ Jr: Basal ganglia calcification as a late radiation effect. AJR 1975;123:27-30

Gamut B-5

CURVILINEAR OR RING-LIKE INTRACRANIAL CALCIFICATION

I. VASCULAR
1. Aneurysm
2. Arteriosclerosis (esp. internal carotid artery)
3. Hemangioma, AV malformation
4. Hematoma

II. NEOPLASTIC
1. Cystic astrocytoma
2. Cystic craniopharyngioma
3. Lipoma of corpus callosum
4. Teratoma, pinealoma

III. PARASITIC
1. Cysticercus cyst (occasionally ring-like calcification)
2. Hydatid cyst
3. Paragonimus cyst (often "soap-bubble" calcification)

CLASSIFICATION OF PRIMARY BRAIN TUMORS

Tumors of Brain and Meninges

I. GLIOMAS
1. Astrocytoma
   a. Astrocytoma, low grade (I and II)
   b. Glioblastoma multiforme (grades III and IV)
2. Oligodendroglioma
3. Paraglioma
   a. Ependymoma
   b. Choroid plexus papilloma or carcinoma
4. Ganglioglioma
5. Medulloblastoma (PNET)

II. PINEAL TUMOR
1. Germinoma
2. Pineoblastoma
3. Pineocytoma
4. Teratoma
5. Teratocarcinoma (embryonal cell carcinoma)

III. PITUITARY TUMOR
1. Adenoma (eosinophilic, basophilic, chromophobe)
2. Carcinoma

IV. MENINGIOMA

V. NERVE SHEATH TUMOR
1. Neurinoma, schwannoma
2. Neurofibroma

VI. MISCELLANEOUS
1. Hemangioblastoma
2. Lipoma (esp. corpus callosum)
3. Sarcoma

Tumors Arising from Embryonal Remnants

1. Colloid cyst
2. Craniopharyngioma
3. Dermoid
4. Epidermoid
5. Teratoma

Reference:
1. Dähnert W: Radiology Review Manual. Baltimore: Williams & Wilkins, 1991, pp 116-117

Subgamut B-6A

INCIDENCE OF BRAIN TUMORS

Classification	Percent Incidence	
	Walker	Lane
Glioblastoma multiforme	23.0	25
Astrocytoma, low grade	13.0	9
Ependymoma	1.8	3
Oligodendroglioma	1.6	2
Mixed & other gliomas	1.9	3
Medulloblastoma (PNET)	1.5	3
Meningioma	16.0	14
Pituitary adenoma	8.2	11
Neurilemoma (esp. acoustic)	5.7	7
Craniopharyngioma	2.8	3
Hemangioblastoma	2.7	
Sarcoma	2.5	
Pineal tumor	1.1	1
Metastatic*	13.0	
Other rare tumors (eg, dermoid, epidermoid, colloid cyst, choroid plexus papilloma)	7.0	3

* Actual incidence of metastatic tumors is higher since more are being identified with CT and MRI, and many others are not worked up radiologically.

References:
1. Lane BA, Moseley IF, Théron J: Intracranial tumors. In: Grainger RG, Allison DJ (eds): Diagnostic Radiology. Edinburgh: Churchill Livingstone, 1992, vol 3, p 1935
2. Walker M: Malignant brain tumors-A synopsis. CA-Cancer J for Clinicians 1975;25:114-120

Gamut B-7

INTRACRANIAL TUMORS IN INFANCY AND CHILDHOOD

Supratentorial Tumors

COMMON
*1. Astrocytoma, cerebral
*2. Choroid plexus papilloma of lateral ventricle
*3. Craniopharyngioma
 4. Optic nerve glioma
*5. Pineal tumor (eg, germinoma, pineoblastoma, pineocytoma, teratoma)

UNCOMMON
 1. Colloid cyst
*2. Ependymoma of third or lateral ventricle
 3. Glioma or hamartoma of hypothalamus
 4. Meningioma; dural sarcoma
 5. Oligodendroglioma
 6. Pituitary adenoma

Infratentorial Tumors

COMMON
*1. Astrocytoma, cerebellar
 2. Brain stem glioma

*3. Ependymoma of fourth ventricle
*4. Medulloblastoma

UNCOMMON
*1. Choroid plexus papilloma of fourth ventricle

* May be present at birth or shortly thereafter.

Gamut B-8

METASTATIC DISEASE TO THE BRAIN AND SKULL (PRIMARY SITES OF ORIGIN)

1. Cerebral parenchymal metastases (esp. from lung, breast, GI or GU tract, or paranasal sinus carcinoma, or melanoma) - seen in approximately 18% of cancer patients
2. Hemorrhagic cerebral parenchymal metastases (esp. melanoma, choriocarcinoma, thyroid, renal cell, lung or breast carcinoma)
3. Meningeal carcinomatosis (8% to 10% of all intra-cranial metastases)
   a. Seeding from primary CNS tumors (eg, medullo-blastoma, ependymoma, pineoblastoma)
   b. Metastatic spread from melanoma, breast or lung cancer
4. Skull metastases
   a. Adult - breast or lung carcinoma; multiple myeloma
   b. Child - neuroblastoma, leukemia

Reference:
1. Sze G (New Haven, CT): Lecture at Hawaii Radiological Society Meeting, 1992

Gamut B-9

SOLITARY INTRACRANIAL MASS

Neoplasm

PRIMARY (CEREBRAL, CEREBELLAR)

1. Congenital
   a. Chordoma
   b. Craniopharyngioma; Rathke's cleft cyst
   c. Dermoid, teratoma
   d. Epidermoid
   e. Hemangioma, hemangioblastoma
   f. Pineal tumor
2. Cranial nerve origin
   a. Acoustic neurinoma
   b. Glioma of optic nerve
   c. Trigeminal neurinoma, other cranial neurinomas
3. Glioma
   a. Low-grade glioma (grade I and II)
   b. Anaplastic astrocytoma (grade III)
   c. Glioblastoma multiforme (grade IV)
   d. Ependymoma, subependymoma
   e. Mixed glioma
   f. Oligodendroglioma
4. Primitive neuroectodermal tumor (PNET)
   a. Supratentorial PNET (cerebral neuroblastoma; pineoblastoma)
   b. Medulloblastoma
   c. Medulloepithelioma
   d. Pigmented medulloblastoma (melanotic vermian PNET)
   e. Ependymoblastoma
5. Pineal tumor
   a. Germinoma
   b. Pineoblastoma
   c. Pineocytoma
   d. Teratoma
   e. Teratocarcinoma

6. Intraventricular
   a. Choroid plexus papilloma or carcinoma
   b. Colloid cyst
   c. Meningioma
7. Lymphoma$_g$ (esp. in AIDS)
8. Meningioma
9. Pituitary tumor
10. Sarcoma

METASTATIC CARCINOMA (ESP. LUNG, BREAST, KIDNEY, MELANOMA)

Nonneoplastic Intracranial Mass

VASCULAR LESION
1. Aneurysm of carotid or vertebral artery or their branches
2. Arteriovenous malformation
3. Cavernous angioma
4. Vein of Galen "aneurysm"

HEMATOMA
1. Epidural
2. Intracerebral (traumatic or spontaneous)
3. Subdural

INFECTION
1. Abscess
   a. Extracerebral
      1. Epidural
      2. Subarachnoid
      3. Subdural
   b. Intracerebral
2. Granulomatous disease
   a. Fungus disease$_g$ (eg, cryptococcosis)
   b. Sarcoidosis

    c. Syphilis
    d. Tuberculosis
3. AIDS and its associated conditions
    a. HIV encephalitis
    b. Progressive multifocal leukoencephalopathy (PML)
    c. Toxoplasmosis
    d. [Lymphoma$_g$]
    e. [Kaposi sarcoma]
    f. Cryptococcosis

INFLAMMATORY CONDITION
1. Tumefactive multiple sclerosis
2. Acute disseminated encephalomyelitis (ADEM)

CYST
1. Dandy-Walker S.
2. Leptomeningeal
3. Parasitic (eg, hydatid, paragonimus, cysticercus, strongyloides)
4. Porencephalic

Gamut B-10

CT ATTENUATION (DENSITY) OF VARIOUS INTRACRANIAL LESIONS (RELATIVE TO NORMAL BRAIN)

Hyperdense

COMMON
1. Acoustic neurinoma
2. Aneurysm, large
3. AV malformation
4. Craniopharyngioma (solid or calcified)
5. Cysticercosis

6. Hematoma (2 weeks old or less) (eg, acute intra-cerebral hemorrhage, acute subdural or epidural hematoma)
7. Medulloblastoma
8. Meningioma
9. Metastasis, hemorrhagic (esp. melanoma, chorio-carcinoma, thyroid, lung, or renal carcinoma); cal-cified metastasis (eg, osteosarcoma, mucinous adenocarcinoma of colon)
10. Pituitary adenoma (esp. chromophobe)

UNCOMMON
1. Choroid plexus papilloma or carcinoma
2. Colloid cyst
3. Ependymoma
4. Glioblastoma multiforme
5. Hamartoma (eg, in tuberous sclerosis)
6. Lymphoma$_g$, primary or secondary
7. Oligodendroglioma
8. Pineoblastoma; pineocytoma; germinoma

Isodense

COMMON
1. Acoustic neurinoma
2. Astrocytoma, low grade or high grade (glioblastoma)
3. Craniopharyngioma (solid or cystic)
4. Hematoma (2 to 4 weeks old)
5. Metastasis
6. Pituitary adenoma

UNCOMMON
1. Chordoma
2. Colloid cyst
3. Ependymoma
4. Ganglioglioma; neuroblastoma
5. Glioma of brain stem

6. Granuloma (esp. tuberculoma)
7. Hemangioblastoma (cystic)
8. Lymphoma$_g$, primary
9. Pineocytoma; germinoma

Hypodense

COMMON

1. Abscess, intracerebral or epidural
2. Astrocytoma, low grade, cystic, or high grade (glioblastoma)
3. Cerebritis (bacterial, tuberculous, fungal)
4. Cyst
   a. Arachnoid
   b. Leptomeningeal
   c. Parasitic (eg, hydatid, paragonimus, cysticercus, strongyloides)
   d. Porencephalic
5. Cystic neoplasm, other
6. Glioma of brain stem
7. Granuloma (esp. tuberculoma)
8. Hematoma, intracerebral or subdural (over 4 weeks old)
9. Infarct, cerebral
10. Metastasis (esp. from squamous cell primary)
11. Multiple sclerosis (periventricular)

UNCOMMON

1. Craniopharyngioma (cystic)
2. Dermoid, teratoma
3. Epidermoid (primary cholesteatoma)
4. Ganglioglioma, ganglioneuroma, neuroblastoma
5. Herpes simplex encephalitis
6. Lipoma
7. Necrosis of globus pallidus (basal ganglia)
8. Prolactinoma
9. Radiation necrosis
10. Subdural empyema

References:
1. Eisenberg RL: Clinical Imaging: An Atlas of Differential Diagnosis. (ed 2) Rockville, MD: Aspen Publishers, 1992
2. Lee SH, Rao K: Cranial Computed Tomography and MRI. (ed 2) New York: McGraw-Hill, 1987, p 314

Gamut B-11

CONTRAST ENHANCEMENT PATTERNS OF INTRACRANIAL MASSES ON CT

Marked Enhancement: Homogeneous

COMMON
1. Aneurysm, large
2. Meningioma
3. Metastasis
4. Pituitary adenoma

UNCOMMON
1. Acoustic neurinoma
2. Choroid plexus papilloma or carcinoma
3. Ependymoma
4. Germinoma, teratocarcinoma (pineal)
5. Hemangioblastoma
6. Lymphoma$_g$, primary or secondary

Marked Enhancement: Patchy, Mixed, or Ring-like

COMMON
1. Astrocytoma, high grade (glioblastoma)
2. AV malformation; large aneurysm
3. Metastasis

UNCOMMON
1. Pineoblastoma

Moderate Enhancement: Variable in Appearance

COMMON
1. Abscess (ring-like)
2. Craniopharyngioma (homogeneous, mixed, or ring-like)
3. Cysticercus cyst (ring-like)
4. Ependymoma (homogeneous or patchy)
5. Granuloma (esp. tuberculoma) (ring-like)
6. Medulloblastoma (homogeneous)

UNCOMMON
1. Chordoma
2. Glomus tumor
3. Hemangioblastoma (homogeneous)
4. Neuroblastoma (mixed)
5. Oligodendroglioma (mixed)
6. Pineocytoma (homogeneous)

Minimal or No Enhancement

COMMON
1. Astrocytoma, low grade (mixed) or cystic (homogeneous)
2. Cyst
   a. Arachnoid
   b. Colloid
   c. Leptomeningeal
   d. Parasitic (eg, hydatid, cysticercus, paragonimus, strongyloides
   e. Porencephalic
3. Hematoma (may show faint ring-like enhancement during resorption - 2 to 6 weeks old)

UNCOMMON

1. Craniopharyngioma, cystic
2. Dermoid, teratoma (no enhancement)
3. Epidermoid (no enhancement)
4. Ganglioglioma (mixed)
5. Lipoma (no enhancement)
6. Prolactinoma (no enhancement)

References:
1. Lange S, Grumme T, Meese W: Computerized Tomography of the Brain. Berlin: Schering Medico-Scientific Book Series, 1980
2. Lee SH, Rao K: Cranial Computed Tomography and MRI. (ed 2) New York: McGraw-Hill, 1987, p 314

VISUAL ESTIMATION OF CT ATTENUATION AND ENHANCEMENT IN VARIOUS SELLAR AND PARASELLAR LESIONS

Type of Lesion	No. of Cases	Attenuation relative to that of brain				Enhancement	
		Higher	Lower	Equal	Mixed	Present	Absent
Craniopharyngioma	11	2		4	5	6	1
Chromophobe adenoma	9	4		2	3	7	
Eosinophilic adenoma	4			2	2	2	
Dermoid cyst	2		2				1
Arachnoid cyst	2		2				1
Meningioma	4	4				4	
Optic glioma	2		1		1	2	
Metastasis	1	1				1	
Aneurysm	2	2				2	
Unverified tumor	2				2	1	
Total	39					25	3

Reference:

1. Hatam A, Bergström M, Greitz T: Diagnosis of sellar and parasellar lesions by computed tomography. Neuroradiology 1979;18: 249–258

Gamut B-13

FEATURES USEFUL IN CT IDENTIFICATION OF VARIOUS TYPES OF NEOPLASM*

Tumor	Initial density	Frequency calcification	Edema	Enhancement pattern	Age/sex group	Location	Other findings
				Extra-axial			
Meningioma	↑	20%	+1	+3 H	A/F	Dural attachment	Occasional hemorrhage
Pineoblastoma	↑	Rare	0	+3 M	P/M	Pineal region	Irregular margin and hypodense center
Choroid plexus papilloma or carcinoma	↑	Rare	0	+3 H	P	Ventricular system	Occasional hemorrhage, irregular margin
Colloid cyst	↑	0	0	0/+1 H	A	Anterior 3d ventricle	
Germinoma	↑/↔	Rare	0	+3 H	A/M	Pineal region	Meningeal and ependymal seeding
Pituitary adenoma	↔/↑	<5%	0	+3 H	A	Sella	Rare hemorrhage or infarction
Neuroma	↔/↑	0	+1	+3 H	A	Cerebellopontine angle	Occasionally cystic
Pineocytoma	↔/↑	Rare	0	+3 H	P	Pineal region	Some cystic
Craniopharyngioma	↔/↓	30/80%	0	+2 M/R	A/P	Suprasellar	Some cystic
Teratoma	↓	Frequent	+1/0	0	P/A/M	Midline supratentorial	Some cystic, rupture, seeding
Dermoid; epidermoid	↓	Frequent	+1/0	0	P/A/F	Post-fossa base of skull	Some cystic
Lipoma	↓	Rare	+1/0	0	P/A	Supratentorial midline	

Tumor	Initial density	Frequency calcification	Edema	Enhancement pattern	Age/sex group	Location	Other findings
				Intra-axial			
Primary lymphoma	↑/↔	0	+2	+2/+3 H	A	Peripheral and deep structures	Irregular margin, multiplicity
Medulloblastoma	↑	10%	+2	+2 H	P	Vermis	Irregular margin
Oligodendroglioma	↑	>90%	+1	+2 M	A	Supratentorial	Irregular margin
Ependymoma	↔/↑	30-40%	+2	+2 H	P	4th ventricle	Irregular margin
Embryonal cell carcinoma	↑/↓	Rare	+1	+3 H	P	Pineal	
Hemangioblastoma	↔/↓	0	+1	+3 H	A	Posterior	Cystic, mural nodule
Ganglioglioma	↓/↔	>30%	0	+1 M	P/A	Temporal lobe	Irregular margin, cystic
Neuroblastoma	↔/↓	Common	+2	+2 M	P	Supratentorial	Hemorrhage
Low-grade astrocytoma	↔/↓	<30%	+1	0/+1 M	A	Supratentorial	Indistinct margin
High-grade astrocytoma (glioblastoma)	↔/↓	Rare	+2	+2-3 M/R	A	Supratentorial	Can be cystic, irregular margin
Brain stem glioma	↓/↔	0	0	+1/M	P	Brain stem	Indistinct margin
Cystic astrocytoma	↓	Rare	+1	+1 H	P	Posterior	Mural tumor nodule

Key: ↑ = Hyperdensity   +1 = Minimal enhancement   H = Homogeneous   A = Adult; P = Pediatric
↔ = Isodensity   +2 = Moderate enhancement   M = Mixed   M = Male predominance
↓ = Hypodensity   +3 = Intense enhancement   R = Ring pattern   F = Female predominance

* This table was prepared by Russell A. Binder, M.D., and S.H. Lee, M.D. in 1982 and modified by S.H. Lee, M.D. in 1986.

Reference:

1. Lee SH, Rao K: Cranial Computed Tomography and MRI. (ed 2), New York: McGraw-Hill, 1987, p 314

Gamut B-14

PINEAL AREA MASS

COMMON
1. Pineal cyst (cystic pineal gland)
2. Pineal tumor (eg, germinoma, pineoblastoma, pineocytoma, teratoma, teratocarcinoma)

UNCOMMON
1. Glioma of nonpineal origin (eg, tumor arising in thalamus, posterior hypothalamus, tectal plate of mesencephalon, or splenium with extension into quadrigeminal cistern)
2. Meningioma
3. Metastasis (midline tumor arising from edge of tentorium)
4. Vein of Galen "aneurysm" (AVM)

Reference:
1. Eisenberg RL: Clinical Imaging: An Atlas of Differential Diagnosis. (ed 2) Rockville, MD: Aspen Publishers, 1992, pp 922-925

Gamut B-15

MIDLINE SUPRATENTORIAL TUMOR OR CYST

Tumors

COMMON
1. Astrocytoma
2. Craniopharyngioma
3. Optic glioma; hypothalamic glioma

4. Pineal tumor (eg, germinoma, pineoblastoma, teratoma) or cyst
5. Pituitary adenoma

UNCOMMON
1. Choroid plexus papilloma or carcinoma
2. Lipoma of corpus callosum
3. Meningioma

Cystic Structures or Lesions

1. Arachnoid cyst
2. Cavum septi pellucidi ("fifth ventricle")
3. Cavum veli interpositi
4. Cavum vergae ("sixth ventricle")
5. Colloid cyst of third ventricle
6. Cystic neoplasm (esp. craniopharyngioma)
7. Parasitic cyst

Reference:

1. Dähnert W: Radiology Review Manual. Baltimore: Williams & Wilkins, 1991, pp 115-117

Gamut B-16

INTRAVENTRICULAR TUMOR OR CYST

COMMON
1. Astrocytoma
2. Colloid cyst (third ventricle)
3. Cysticercosis
4. Ependymoma
5. Meningioma

UNCOMMON
1. Arachnoid cyst
2. AV malformation
3. Choroid plexus papilloma or carcinoma
4. Craniopharyngioma (third ventricle)
5. Dermoid, teratoma
6. Epidermoid
7. Medulloblastoma
8. Metastasis
9. Subependymoma

Gamut B-17

VENTRICULAR WALL NODULE(S)

COMMON
*1. Choroid plexus
2. Heterotopic gray matter
3. Nodular caudate nucleus
*4. Tuberous sclerosis

UNCOMMON
1. Coarctation of lateral ventricles with ependymal adhesions
*2. Cysticercosis
3. Ependymal seeding from malignant brain tumor (eg, ependymoma, medulloblastoma, glioblastoma)
4. Ependymitis (esp. torulosis)
5. Intraventricular neoplasm (eg, ependymoma, subependymoma, epidermoid, meningioma, choroid plexus papilloma or carcinoma)

* May show calcification.

Reference:
1. Bergeron RT: Pneumographic demonstration of subependymal heterotopic cortical gray matter in children. AJR 1967; 101:168-177

Gamut B-18

WIDENING OF THE SEPTUM PELLUCIDUM (GREATER THAN 3 MM)

COMMON
1. Cyst or neoplasm of septum pellucidum
2. Noncommunicating cavum septi pellucidi

UNCOMMON
1. Corpus callosum neoplasm infiltrating septum pellucidum
2. Intraventricular astrocytoma extending into septum pellucidum
3. Lipoma of corpus callosum
4. Neoplasm of third ventricle

Gamut B-19

MASS INVOLVING THE POSTERIOR PORTION OF THE THIRD VENTRICLE

COMMON
1. Cystic pineal gland
2. Ependymoma
3. Glioma or other neoplasm arising from quadri-geminal body
4. Pinealoma, teratoma

UNCOMMON
1. Meningioma (eg, intraventricular or incisural)
2. Quadrigeminal cyst
3. Vein of Galen "aneurysm" (AVM)

Gamut B-20

INFRATENTORIAL LESIONS (FOURTH VENTRICLE, CEREBELLAR, AND OTHER POSTERIOR FOSSA LESIONS) (See Gamuts B-21 to B-27)

Fourth Ventricle (Intraventricular) Lesions

COMMON
1. Ependymoma

UNCOMMON
1. Angioma
2. Choroid plexus papilloma or carcinoma
3. Cysticercosis
4. Dermoid; epidermoid
5. Meningioma
6. Metastasis
7. Subependymoma

Cerebellar (Parenchymal) Lesions

COMMON
1. Astrocytoma
2. Hemangioblastoma (esp. in von Hippel-Lindau disease)
3. Hemorrhage
4. Infarction
5. Infection, abscess (eg, pyogenic, tuberculous, fungal); cysticercosis; sarcoidosis
6. Medulloblastoma, other PNET (See B-21)
7. Metastasis

UNCOMMON
1. Dysplastic gangliocytoma of cerebellum - purkingeoma (Lhermitte-Duclos disease)
2. Lymphoma$_g$
3. Sarcoma (lateral medulloblastoma)

B. Brain   33

Other Posterior Fossa (Extra-axial) Lesions

COMMON

1. Aneurysm of basilar artery
2. Aqueductal stenosis (eg, from midbrain glioma)
3. Cerebellopontine angle neoplasm (eg, acoustic neurinoma, meningioma, epidermoid) (See B-26)
4. Chordoma of clivus
5. Glioma (astrocytoma) of brain stem (pons)

UNCOMMON

1. Arteriovenous malformation

References:

1. Bundschuh CV: Posterior fossa abnormalities on 0.3 tesla MRI scanner. Radiological Society of North America Scientific Exhibit, Washington, D.C., 1984
2. Damiano T, Truwit CL: Cerebellar and fourth ventricular tumors in adults. MRI Decisions 1992;6:10-21
3. Eisenberg RL: Clinical Imaging: An Atlas of Differential Diagnosis. (ed 2) Rockville, MD: Aspen Publishers, 1992, pp 900-911

Gamut B-21

POSTERIOR FOSSA TUMORS IN CHILDREN (OVER 1 YEAR OF AGE) ON CT OR MRI

COMMON

1. Cerebellar astrocytoma (juvenile pilocytic)
2. Ependymoma
3. Primitive neuroectodermal tumor (PNET)
    a. Cerebellar medulloblastoma
    b. Ependymoblastoma
    c. Medulloepithelioma
    d. Pigmented medulloblastoma (melanotic vermian PNET)

UNCOMMON
1. Acoustic neurinoma (esp. with neurofibromatosis)
2. Brain stem astrocytoma
3. Cavernous hemangioma
4. Dysplastic gangliocytoma of cerebellum (Lhermitte-Duclos disease)
5. Hemangioblastoma (rare below age 15)
6. Rhabdosarcoma

References:

1. Atlas SW: Magnetic Resonance Imaging of the Brain and Spine. New York: Raven Press, 1991
2. Fitz CR, Rao K: Primary tumors in children. In: Lee SH, Rao K: Cranial Computed Tomography and MRI. (ed 2) New York: McGraw-Hill, 1987, pp 365-381

Gamut B-22

CYSTIC OR NECROTIC MASS IN THE POSTERIOR FOSSA (AS SEEN ON CT, MRI, OR ULTRASOUND)

CONGENITAL CRANIOCEREBRAL MASS OR MALFORMATION
1. Dandy-Walker cyst
2. Ependymal cyst
3. Extra-axial arachnoid cyst
4. Giant cisterna magna

INFECTIOUS LESION
1. Abscess (esp. streptococcal, anaerobic)
2. Granulomatous infection (tuberculosis or fungus disease$_g$)
3. Parasitic disease$_g$ (eg, cysticercosis, hydatid disease, paragonimiasis)

BENIGN OR MALIGNANT NEOPLASM

1. Acoustic neurinoma with associated arachnoid cyst (about 5%)
2. Brain stem glioma
3. Cystic astrocytoma
4. Ependymoma
5. Epidermoid, dermoid
6. Hemangioblastoma
7. Medulloblastoma (rarely tiny cystic areas)
8. Metastasis
9. [Tumefactive multiple sclerosis]

TRAPPED FOURTH VENTRICLE (POSTSHUNTING)

Reference:

1. Batnitzky S, Price HI, Gilmor RL: Cystic lesions of the posterior fossa. Radiological Society of North America Scientific Exhibit, Washington, 1984

Gamut B-23

OBSTRUCTION AT THE FOURTH VENTRICLE OUTLET[*]

COMMON

1. Atresia of fourth ventricle foramina (eg, Dandy-Walker S.)
2. Basilar arachnoiditis (eg, tuberculous meningitis)
3. Basilar invagination (eg, Paget's disease)
4. Chiari I and Chiari II (Arnold-Chiari) malformations
5. Neoplasm (esp. medulloblastoma, astrocytoma, ependymoma, metastasis)
6. Tonsillar herniation

UNCOMMON

1. Congenital arachnoid cyst
2. Cysticercus cyst

3. Fusion deformity at craniovertebral junction
4. Meningocele

* Enlargement of the entire ventricular system with disproportionate dilatation of the fourth ventricle.

Gamut B-24

ENLARGED BRAIN STEM

COMMON
1. Glioma
2. Hemorrhage
3. Metastatic neoplasm

UNCOMMON
1. Abscess
2. Encephalitis
3. Ependymoma
4. Granulomatous disease (eg, sarcoidosis, tuberculosis)
5. Hemangioblastoma
6. Infarction, acute
7. Medulloblastoma
8. Other tumors (eg, lipoma, hamartoma, teratoma, epidermoid, lymphoma)
9. Syringobulbia
10. Vascular anomaly

References:
1. Ball JB: Enlarged brain stem. Semin Roentgenol 1984;19:3-4
2. Harwood-Nash DCF, Fitz CR: Neuroradiology in Infants and Children. St. Louis: C.V. Mosby, 1976, vol 2, pp 718-724

Gamut B-25

LOW ATTENUATION (HYPODENSE) LESION IN THE BRAIN STEM ON CT

COMMON
1. Glioma
2. Infarction
3. Metastasis
4. Multiple sclerosis

UNCOMMON
1. Central pontine myelinosis
2. Epidermoid
3. Granuloma, abscess (eg, tuberculosis or other infection; sarcoidosis)
4. Hamartoma
5. Lipoma
6. Lymphoma$_g$
7. Syringobulbia
8. Teratoma

Reference:
1. Eisenberg RL: Clinical Imaging: An Atlas of Differential Diagnosis. (ed 2) Rockville, MD: Aspen Publishers, 1992, pp 934-935

Gamut B-26

CEREBELLOPONTINE ANGLE MASS

COMMON
1. Acoustic neurinoma
2. Arachnoid cyst
3. Basilar or vertebral artery aneurysm or ectasia
4. Epidermoid (primary cholesteatoma)
5. Meningioma
6. Pontine glioma, fourth ventricular tumor, or cerebellar neoplasm (eg, astrocytoma, hemangioblastoma) with lateral extension

UNCOMMON

1. AV malformation
2. Chordoma
3. Glomus jugulare tumor
4. Metastasis
5. Other neurinoma (VII, X, XI or XII nerve)
6. [Parasellar neoplasm with extension (eg, chromophobe adenoma, optic glioma, craniopharyngioma, nasopharyngeal carcinoma)]
7. Rhabdomyosarcoma

References:

1. Eisenberg RL: Clinical Imaging: An Atlas of Differential Diagnosis. (ed 2) Rockville, MD: Aspen Publishers, 1992, pp 926-933
2. Newton TH, Potts DG: Radiology of the Skull and Brain. St. Louis: C.V. Mosby, 1971, vol 1, book 1, pp 442-447
3. Smoker WR, Jacoby CG, Mojtahedi S, et al: The CT gamut of cerebellopontine angle lesions. Radiological Society of North America Scientific Exhibit, Washington, 1984

Gamut B-27

MASS IN THE CLIVUS OR PREPONTINE AREA

COMMON

1. Aneurysm of basilar or vertebral artery
2. Chordoma
3. Meningioma

UNCOMMON

1. Bone sarcoma (esp. chondrosarcoma, osteosarcoma)
2. Epidermoid
3. Metastasis
4. Nasopharyngeal neoplasm with extension
5. Osteochondroma
6. Parasellar neoplasm with extension (eg, craniopharyngioma, optic glioma, chromophobe adenoma)

MASS IN THE MIDDLE FOSSA
(See Gamuts C-27, C-28)

COMMON

1. Aneurysm of internal carotid artery (large); carotid-cavernous fistula
2. Arachnoid cyst
3. Intra-axial temporal lobe neoplasm, hematoma, or abscess
4. Meningioma of sphenoid ridge or middle fossa
5. Nasopharyngeal or paranasal sinus carcinoma or other neoplasm with middle fossa extension
6. Subdural hematoma

UNCOMMON

1. Epidermoid (cholesteatoma)
2. Histiocytosis X_g
3. Metastasis
4. Midline neoplasm extending laterally (eg, chordoma, craniopharyngioma, pituitary adenoma)
5. Neurinoma (eg, fifth nerve, gasserian ganglion)

References:

1. DuBoulay GH: Principles of X-ray Diagnosis of the Skull. (ed 2) London: Butterworths, 1980
2. Newton TH, Potts DG: Radiology of the Skull and Brain. St. Louis: C.V. Mosby, 1971, vol 1, book 1, pp 311-313

Gamut B-29

MULTIPLE ENHANCING LESIONS IN THE CEREBRUM AND CEREBELLUM ON CT

COMMON
1. Metastasis (esp. from lung, breast, colon, rectum, or kidney carcinoma, or melanoma)
2. Multifocal infectious disease (eg, tuberculosis, histoplasmosis)
3. Multiple sclerosis (periventricular)
4. Parasitic disease (eg, cysticercosis, toxoplasmosis)

UNCOMMON
1. AV malformations, aneurysms
2. Infarction, subacute multifocal
    a. Arterial (eg, underperfusion; multiple emboli; cerebral vasculitis due to lupus erythematosus; meningitis)
    b. Venous (superior sagittal sinus thrombosis with parasagittal hemorrhages)
3. Lymphoma$_g$, primary (esp. in immunosuppressed or organ transplant patients)
4. Sarcoidosis (usually in meninges)

Reference:
1. Eisenberg RL: Clinical Imaging: An Atlas of Differential Diagnosis. Rockville, MD: Aspen Publishers, 1992, pp 908-911

Gamut B-30

RING-ENHANCING LESION ON CT

COMMON
1. Abscess
2. Glioblastoma multiforme

---

3. Hematoma, intracerebral (3-6 weeks old)
4. Lymphoma$_g$ (esp. in transplant recipients or in AIDS)
5. Metastasis
6. Subdural hematoma, resolving (1 to 4 weeks old)

UNCOMMON
1. Aneurysm, large (occasionally)
2. Craniopharyngioma
3. Cysticercus cyst
4. Granuloma (esp. tuberculoma)
5. Meningioma (atypical)
6. Radiation necrosis

References:
1. Eisenberg RL: Clinical Imaging: An Atlas of Differential Diagnosis. (ed 2) Rockville, MD: Aspen Publishers, 1992, pp 896-899
2. Lee SH, Rao K: Cranial Computed Tomography and MRI. (ed 2) New York: McGraw-Hill, 1987, p 314

Gamut B-31

SURFACE ENHANCEMENT OF THE BRAIN ON CT

I. RIM OR LINEAR ENHANCEMENT (INDICATES ABNORMAL FLUID COLLECTION OVER BRAIN SURFACE)
1. Empyema, subdural or epidural
2. Hematoma, subdural or epidural

II. DIFFUSE GYRIFORM ENHANCEMENT (INDICATES DISSEMINATED MENINGEAL DISEASE)
1. Lymphoma$_g$, leukemia
2. Meningeal carcinomatosis (eg, from breast, lung, melanoma)
3. Meningitis (eg, pyogenic, tuberculous, fungal, viral, sarcoid)

4. Neoplastic seeding from primary CNS tumor (ependymoma, medulloblastoma, pineoblastoma)
5. Subarachnoid hemorrhage, late (with fibroblastic proliferation)

III. LOCALIZED GYRIFORM ENHANCEMENT
1. AV malformation
*2. Encephalitis
*3. Infarction
*4. Glioma

IV. BASILAR CISTERN ENHANCEMENT
1. Meningeal neoplasms
2. Torulosis (cryptococcosis)
3. Tuberculous meningitis

* Parenchymal lesions which infiltrate the cortex and obliterate the sulci.

References:
1. Burrows EH: Surface enhancement of the brain. Clin Radiol 1985;36:233-239
2. Chapman S, Nakielny R: Aids to Radiological Differential Diagnosis. (ed 2) London:Baillière Tindall, 1990, p 350

Gamut B-32

ENHANCING VENTRICULAR MARGINS ON CT

COMMON
1. Meningeal carcinomatosis (esp. from lung, breast, melanoma)
2. Subependymal or ependymal spread of primary brain neoplasm (esp. glioma, ependymoma, medulloblastoma, germinoma)
3. Ventriculitis, inflammatory (eg, bacterial, fungal, or parasitic infection - esp. cysticercosis); sarcoidosis

UNCOMMON
1. Leukemia
2. Lymphoma, primary or systemic

Reference:
1. Eisenberg RL: Clinical Imaging: An Atlas of Differential Diagnosis. Rockville, MD: Aspen Publishers, 1992, pp 944-945

Gamut B-33

INCREASED DENSITY WITHIN THE BASILAR CISTERNS ON THE NONENHANCED CT SCAN

COMMON
1. Iodinated intrathecal contrast
2. Subarachnoid hemorrhage

UNCOMMON
1. Basilar cistern infection, active (eg, tuberculosis, cryptococcosis, coccidiomycosis)
2. Bromism
3. En plaque neoplasm (eg, lymphoma$_g$, melanoma, meningioma)
4. Epidermoid
5. Meningeal calcification (eg, prior tuberculosis)
6. Polycythemia
7. Postischemic hypervascularity of the meninges
8. Sarcoidosis

References:
1. Enzmann DR: Imaging of Infections and Inflammations of the CNS: CT, Ultrasound and NMR. New York: Raven Press, 1984
2. Holmes S: Personal communication
3. Lee SH, Rao K: Cranial Computed Tomography and MRI. (ed 2) New York: McGraw-Hill, 1987

B. Brain

4. Masdeau JC, Fine M, Shewmon DA, et al: Post-ischemic hypervascularity of the infant brain: Differential diagnosis on CT. AJNR 1982;3:501-544
5. Osborne DDR, Bohan T, Hudson A: CT demonstration of hyperdense cerebral vasculature due to bromide therapy. J Comput Assist Tomogr 1984;8:982-984
6. Pagani JJ, Libshitz HI, Wallace S: CNS leukemia and lymphoma: CT manifestations. AJNR 1981;2:397-403

Gamut B-34

INTENSE ENHANCEMENT OF THE BASILAR CISTERNS ON CT

COMMON

1. Leptomeningeal neoplasm (eg, carcinomatosis, gliomatosis, lymphoma$_g$, melanoma, seeding from medulloblastoma or other CNS neoplasm)
2. Meningitis
3. Subarachnoid hemorrhage, recent

UNCOMMON

1. Polycythemia vera
2. Sarcoidosis
3. Siderosis
4. Syphilis

References:
1. Enzmann DR: Imaging of Infections and Inflammations of the CNS: CT, Ultrasound and NMR. New York: Raven Press, 1984
2. Holmes S: Personal communication
3. Kudel TA, Bingham WT, Tubman DE: CT findings of primary malignant leptomeningeal melanoma in neurocutaneous melanosis. AJR 1979;133:950-951
4. Pagani JJ, Libshitz HI, Wallace S: CNS leukemia and lymphoma: CT manifestations. AJNR 1981;2:397-403
5. Pinkston JW, Ballinger WE Jr, Lotz PR, et al: Superficial siderosis: A cause of leptomeningeal enhancement on computed tomography. J Comput Assist Tomogr 1983;7:1073-1076

Gamut B-35

INTRACRANIAL FAT OR AIR LUCENCY (ON PLAIN FILMS, CT, OR MRI)

Fat Lucency

COMMON
1. Lipoma of corpus callosum

UNCOMMON
1. Dermoid cyst
2. Epidermoid cyst

Air Lucency (Pneumocephalus)

COMMON
1. Trauma (eg, penetrating injury or fracture of a paranasal sinus or mastoid sinus)

UNCOMMON
1. Air embolism in cerebral vessels
2. Iatrogenic (eg, surgery, pneumoencephalography, ventriculography)
3. Infection with gas-forming organism (brain abscess)
4. Neoplasm of base of skull (esp. osteoma, carcinoma) invading a sinus

References:
1. Azar-Kia B, Sarwar M, Batnitzky S, et al: Radiology of the intracranial gas. AJR 1975;124:315-323
2. Kushnet MW, Goldman RL: Lipoma of the corpus callosum associated with a frontal bone defect. AJR 1978;131:517-518
3. Swischuk LE: Differential Diagnosis in Pediatric Radiology. Baltimore: Williams & Wilkins, 1984, p 378

Gamut B-36

INFECTIONS OF THE BRAIN IDENTIFIABLE ON CT OR MRI

I. FOCAL PARENCHYMAL LESIONS
1. Abscess secondary to emboli
2. Cerebritis
3. Direct extension from sinusitis
4. Trauma with penetrating injury

II. CYSTIC PARASITIC LESIONS
1. Cysticercosis (parenchymal, intraventricular, subarachnoid)
2. Hydatid disease
3. Paragonimiasis

III. DIFFUSE PARENCHYMAL INFECTIONS
1. ADEM, slow viruses
2. AIDS encephalopathy
3. Ebstein-Barr encephalitis
4. Herpes simplex encephalitis
5. Progressive multifocal leukoencephalopathy (PML)

IV. MENINGITIS, EPENDYMITIS (eg, BACTERIAL, VIRAL, TUBERCULOUS)

V. EXTRACEREBRAL INFECTIONS - SUBDURAL OR EPIDURAL EMPYEMA
1. Postmeningitis
2. Posttraumatic
3. Secondary to hematogenous or adjacent spread (eg, from sinusitis)

VI. VASCULITIS SECONDARY TO INFECTION
1. Bacterial
2. Granulomatous (eg, tuberculous, fungal$_g$)
3. Viral (eg, herpes zoster ophthalmicus)

VII. SARCOIDOSIS (DURAL, LEPTOMENINGEAL, INTRAPARENCHYMAL)

Reference:
1. Sze G: Lecture at Hawaii Radiological Society Meeting, 1992

Gamut B-37

WHITE MATTER DISEASE OF THE BRAIN ON CT OR MRI (DEMYELINATING OR DYSMYELINATING DISEASES)

Demyelinating (Myelinoclastic) Diseases (Normal Myelin Is Destroyed)

COMMON
1. Multiple sclerosis
2. Progressive multifocal leukoencephalopathy (PML)

UNCOMMON
1. Acute disseminated encephalomyelitis (ADE)
   a. Allergic (postvaccination)
   b. Fulminating (fatal)
   c. Postinfection (measles, vaccinia, varicella)
   d. Spontaneous or during a respiratory infection
2. Central pontine myelinolysis
3. Disseminated necrotizing leukoencephalopathy (after methotrexate therapy)
4. Marchiafava-Bignami disease (corpus callosum)
5. Schilder's disease (diffuse sclerosis)

Dysmyelinating Diseases
(Abnormal Myelin Formation or Maintenance In Infants and Children)

COMMON
1. Metachromatic leukodystrophy

UNCOMMON
1. Adrenoleukodystrophy
2. Alexander's disease
3. Globoid cell leukodystrophy (Krabbe's disease)
4. Pelizaeus-Merzbacher disease
5. Spongy degeneration (Canavan's disease)

Secondary Demyelinating Conditions

1. Anoxia
2. Brain abscess
3. Cerebral infarct
4. Cerebral neoplasm, primary or metastatic
5. Deficiency syndromes
6. Intoxication

Reference:
1. Lee SH, Rao K: Cranial Computed Tomography and MRI. (ed 2) New York: McGraw-Hill, 1987, pp 717-745

Gamut B-38

CEREBRAL INFARCTION (STROKE) ON CT, MRI, OR ANGIOGRAPHY

I. ARTERIAL OCCLUSIVE DISEASE

1. Arteriolosclerosis (intracerebral arteriolar occlusive disease, esp. with chronic hypertension)
2. Atherosclerotic occlusion of a major artery
3. Embolism (often with hemorrhagic infarction)
4. Hemodynamic ischemia (eg, severe stenosis or chronic occlusion of an artery)
5. Moyamoya disease
6. Vasculitis, arteritis

II. ANOXIC ISCHEMIC ENCEPHALOPATHY DUE TO ACUTE RESPIRATORY INSUFFICIENCY

1. Allergic reaction
2. Carbon monoxide intoxication
3. Cardiac failure or hypotension, acute
4. Drowning
5. Drug overdose (eg, central respiratory depressant drugs, esp. alcohol, narcotics, and barbiturates)
6. Primary central respiratory failure

III. VENOUS THROMBOSIS, SEPTIC OR ASEPTIC (INVOLVING MAJOR VENOUS SINUSES, SUPERFICIAL CORTICAL VEINS, AND/OR DEEP VENOUS SYSTEM)

Reference:
1. Lee SH, Rao K: Cranial Computed Tomography and MRI. (ed 2) New York: McGraw-Hill, 1987, pp 643-699

Gamut B-39

INTRACEREBRAL HEMORRHAGE OR HEMATOMA ON CT, MRI, OR ANGIOGRAPHY

COMMON

1. AV malformation, venous angioma, cavernous angioma
2. Head trauma
3. Hemorrhagic arterial or venous infarction (eg, superior sagittal sinus thrombosis)
4. Neoplasm
5. Rupture of berry or mycotic aneurysm

UNCOMMON

1. Amphetamine abuse
2. Amyloid angiopathy
3. Arteritis
4. Bleeding or clotting disorder
5. Hypertensive vascular disease (arteriolosclerosis)
6. Neonatal germinal matrix hemorrhage (esp. in prematures less than 1500 gm)
7. Surgery

References:

1. Buonanno FS, Moody DM, Ball MR, et al: Computed cranial tomographic findings in cerebral sinovenous occlusion. J Comput Assist Tomogr 1978;2:281-290
2. Harrington H, Heller A, Dawson D, et al: Intracerebral hemorrhage and oral amphetamine. Arch Neurol 1983;40: 503-507
3. Hickey WF, King RB, Wang AM, et al: Multiple simultaneous intracerebral hematomas: Clinical, radiologic and pathologic findings in two patients. Arch Neurol 1983;40: 519-522
4. Holmes S: Personal communication
5. Lee SH, Rao K: Cranial Computed Tomography and MRI. (ed 2) New York: McGraw-Hill, 1987, pp 645, 699-708
6. Wagle WA, Smith TW, Weiner M: Intracerebral hemorrhage caused by cerebral amyloid angiopathy: Radiographic-pathologic correlation. AJNR 1984;5:171-176

Gamut B-40

SUBDURAL EMPYEMA ON CT OR MRI

COMMON
1. Sinusitis (frontal or ethmoid) with spread to subdural space
2. Trauma with penetrating injury to skull

UNCOMMON
1. Mastoiditis, middle ear infection
2. Osteomyelitis of skull
3. Purulent meningitis
4. Surgery (craniectomy)

Reference:
1. Eisenberg RL: Clinical Imaging: An Atlas of Differential Diagnosis. (ed 2) Rockville, MD: Aspen Publishers, 1992, p 884

Gamut B-41

PATTERN ANALYSIS OF CEREBRAL VESSELS ON ANGIOGRAPHY (FILLING, SIZE, NUMBER, CONTOUR, AND TRANSIT TIME)
(See Gamut B-42)

LACK OF VASCULAR FILLING
1. Compression
2. Dissection
3. Embolization (incl. iatrogenic)
4. Shunt
5. Thrombosis (eg, atherosclerosis, vasculitis)

HYPERVASCULARITY (TOO MANY VESSELS)
1. Arteriovenous malformation, vein of Galen aneurysm
2. Collateral circulation
3. Congenital variant
4. Neoplasm

INCREASED SIZE OF VESSELS
1. Aneurysm (incl. vein of Galen)
2. Arteriovenous malformation
3. Carotid - cavernous fistula
4. Ectasia
5. High flow system
6. Neoplasm

DECREASED SIZE OF VESSELS
1. Atherosclerosis
2. Dissection
3. Low flow system
4. Spasm (eg, subarachnoid hemorrhage; migraine)
5. Vasculitis

CONTOUR IRREGULARITY OF VESSEL WALLS
1. Atherosclerosis
2. Dissection
3. Fibromuscular hyperplasia
4. Spasm
5. Tumor vascularity or encasement
6. Vasculitis

PROLONGED TRANSIT TIME
1. Focal edema
2. Hyperventilation, decreased pCO_2
3. Infarction or occlusion
4. Venous thrombosis

DECREASED TRANSIT TIME AND EARLY VENOUS FILLING
1. Arteriovenous malformation
2. Increased pCO_2
3. Infarction
4. Neoplasm

References:
1. Djang WT: Basics of Cerebral Angiography. In: Ravin CE, Cooper C (eds): Review of Radiology. Philadelphia: W.B. Saunders, 1990, pp 189-191
2. Osborne A: Introduction to Cerebral Angiography. Hagerstown, MD: Harper & Row, 1980

ARTERITIS AND OTHER CEREBRAL ARTERIAL DISEASE ON ANGIOGRAPHY (NARROWING, IRREGULARITY, OCCLUSION, OR ANEURYSM)

ARTERITIS

1. Bacterial arteritis, mycotic aneurysm (eg, from abscess, meningitis, osteomyelitis, embolism)
2. Behcet S.
3. Carotid arteritis (infant or child)
4. Collagen disease arteritis (esp. lupus erythematosus)
5. Drug or chemical arteritis (eg, ergot, amphetamine, heroin, arsenic, carbon monoxide)
6. Fungal arteritis (esp. torulosis, actinomycosis, nocardiosis, aspergillosis, phycomycosis)
7. Necrotizing angiitis (eg, polyarteritis nodosa, rheumatic fever, hypersensitivity angiitis, giant cell arteritis, temporal arteritis)
8. Radiation arteritis
9. Rickettsial arteritis
10. Sarcoid arteritis
11. Syphilitic arteritis
12. Takayasu's arteritis
13. Tuberculous arteritis
14. Viral arteritis (eg, herpes zoster)

OTHER CAUSES

1. Arterial spasm (eg, subarachnoid or cerebral hemorrhage; migraine)
2. Arteriosclerosis
3. AV malformation
4. Berry aneurysm
5. Cerebral thrombosis (eg, sickle cell anemia, oral contraceptives)

6. Embolism (eg, subacute bacterial endocarditis, atrial myxoma)
7. Fibromuscular dysplasia (usually extracranial)
8. Idiopathic
9. [Increased intracranial pressure]
10. Inflammatory disease of brain (eg, abscess; purulent or tuberculous meningitis)
11. Multiple progressive intracranial artery occlusions with telangiectasia (moyamoya)
12. Neoplasm (eg, glioblastoma, lymphoma$_g$, metastasis)
13. Neurocutaneous syndromes (eg, neurofibromatosis, Sturge-Weber S., tuberous sclerosis)
14. Trauma

References:

1. Ferris EJ, Levine HL: Cerebral arteritis: Classification. Radiology 1973;109:327-341
2. Grainger RG, Allison DJ (eds): Diagnostic Radiology: An Anglo-American Textbook of Imaging. (ed 2) Edinburgh: Churchill Livingstone, 1992, vol 3, pp 1993-1994
3. Hilal SK, Solomon GE, Gold AP, et al: Primary cerebral arterial occlusive disease in children. Radiology 1971;99: 71-94
4. Leeds NE, Rosenblatt R: Arterial wall irregularities in intracranial neoplasms. Radiology 1972;103:121-124

Gamut B-43

INTRACRANIAL ARTERIOVENOUS SHUNTING AND EARLY VENOUS FILLING ON CEREBRAL ANGIOGRAPHY

COMMON

1. AV malformation, congenital or acquired (incl. carotid-cavernous fistula, vein of Galen "aneurysm")
2. Infarction of brain
3. Occlusive vascular disease
4. Malignant neoplasm of brain, primary or metastatic

UNCOMMON
1. Cerebral arteritis
2. Contusion of brain
3. Epilepsy, focal idiopathic
4. Inflammatory lesion (eg, brain abscess)
5. Intracerebral hematoma

References:

1. Glickman MG, Mainzer F, Gletne JS: Early venous opacification in cerebral contusion. Radiology 1971;100:615-622
2. Lee SH, Goldberg HI: Hypervascular pattern associated with idiopathic focal status epilepticus. Radiology 1977; 125:159-163

Gamut B-44

AVASCULAR ZONE NEAR THE BRAIN SURFACE ON CEREBRAL ANGIOGRAPHY

COMMON
1. Cortical atrophy
2. "Cortical steal" by deep AV shunt
3. Epidural hematoma, hygroma, or empyema
4. Meningeal neoplasm (eg, avascular meningioma; meningeal involvement by carcinoma, lymphoma$_g$, leukemia, sarcoma, neuroblastoma, or melanoma)
5. Occlusive vascular disease; brain infarct
6. Subdural hematoma, hygroma, or empyema

UNCOMMON
1. Arachnoid cyst
2. Bone lesion infiltrating dura (eg, metastasis, sarcoma, epidermoid, histiocytosis X$_g$)
3. Normal large subarachnoid space (infant)
4. Parasitic cyst (eg, cysticercus, hydatid, paragonimus)

5. Porencephalic cyst
6. Subdural invasion by glioma
7. Syphilitic pachymeningitis
8. Tuberculoma

Reference:
1. Ferris EJ, Lehrer H, Shapiro JH: Pseudo-subdural hematoma. Radiology 1967;88:75-84

Gamut B-45

EXTRACRANIAL ISCHEMIC LESION SECONDARILY INVOLVING THE BRAIN

COMMON
1. Occlusion or stenosis of brachiocephalic vessels
2. Steal syndromes (eg, subclavian steal) (See B-46)

UNCOMMON
1. Dissecting aneurysm of thoracic aorta
2. Embolization secondary to mitral valve disease or atrial myxoma
3. Takayasu's arteritis
4. Trauma to neck
5. Tumor in neck compromising cervical vessels (eg, thyroid adenoma, neurilemoma)

Reference:
1. Mishkin MM: Extracranial ischemic lesions which secondarily involve the brain. Radiol Clin North Am 1967;5:395-408

Gamut B-46

SUBCLAVIAN STEAL SYNDROME

COMMON
1. Atherosclerosis

UNCOMMON
1. Coarctation of aorta with obliteration of subclavian orifice
2. Extravascular obstruction (eg, fibrous band)
3. Hypoplasia, atresia, or isolation of subclavian artery with anomalous aortic arch
4. Ligation for correction of tetralogy of Fallot or coarctation of aorta
5. Obstruction of subclavian artery secondary to cannulation
6. Vascular ring

References:
1. Becker AE, Becker MJ, Edwards JE, et al: Congenital anatomic potentials for subclavian steal. Chest 1971;60:4-13
2. Massumi RA: The congenital variety of the subclavian steal syndrome. Circulation 1963;28:1149-1152
3. Patel A, Toole JF: Subclavian steal syndrome: Reversal of cephalic blood flow. Medicine 1965;44:289-303

Gamut B-47

INCREASED INTRACRANIAL PRESSURE

COMMON
1. Brain abscess
2. Cerebral edema, contusion, hemorrhage, or infarction
3. Hematoma (intracerebral, extradural, subdural); hygroma
4. Hydrocephalus, obstructive (See B-48)
5. Lead encephalopathy

6. Meningitis, meningoencephalitis (eg, tuberculosis, torulosis, toxoplasmosis)
7. Metastatic neoplasm (eg, bronchogenic carcinoma, neuroblastoma)
8. Primary brain tumor

UNCOMMON
1. Aqueduct stenosis
2. Arnold-Chiari malformation
3. Craniostenosis, severe
4. Dandy-Walker S.
5. Drug therapy (eg, tetracycline)
6. Emphysema, severe with cough
7. Hyperthyroidism
8. Hypervitaminosis A
9. Hypoparathyroidism
10. Leukemia, lymphoma$_g$
11. Meningocele
12. Parasitic disease (eg, cysticercosis, hydatid disease, paragonimiasis)
13. Pseudotumor cerebri

Subgamut B-47A

RADIOLOGIC FEATURES OF INCREASED INTRACRANIAL PRESSURE

1. Increased craniofacial ratio
2. Increased digital markings of calvarium ("hammered silver" appearance)
3. Sellar changes
   a. Decalcification of floor and dorsum of sella
   b. Pointed anterior clinoids
   c. Sellar enlargement
   d. Thinning or loss of posterior clinoids
4. Sutural diastasis; unusually deep sutural interdigitations
5. Thinning of calvarium

Gamut B-48

HYDROCEPHALUS
(See Subgamuts M-48A, M-48B)

**ATROPHIC HYDROCEPHALUS
(CEREBRAL ATROPHY)**

1. AV malformation, vascular lesion
2. Cerebral maldevelopment (eg, lissencephaly, atrophy of one cerebral hemisphere - Davidoff-Dyke S.)
3. Congenital inflammatory disease (eg, toxoplasmosis, torulosis, cytomegalic inclusion disease)
4. Demyelinating disease (eg, multiple sclerosis, encephalomyelitis)
5. Drugs (eg, Dilantin, steroids, chemotherapy, marijuana, hard drugs); alcohol
6. Hypertensive cerebral degenerative disease
7. Idiopathic
8. Multi-infarct dementia
9. Normal aging
10. Primary neuronal degeneration (eg, Alzheimer's disease, Pick's disease, Jakob-Creutzfeldt disease, Huntington's chorea)
11. Radiation therapy
12. Trauma

**COMMUNICATING HYDROCEPHALUS
SECONDARY TO OBSTRUCTION OF
SUBARACHNOID SPACES AT CEREBRAL
CONVEXITY, BASAL CISTERNS, OR FORAMEN
MAGNUM**

1. Achondroplasia
2. Arnold-Chiari malformation
3. Basilar invagination (See C-10)
4. Encephalocele
5. Meningeal infiltration in storage diseases
6. Meningitis
7. Meningomyelocele
8. Neoplasm

9. Subarachnoid or subdural hemorrhage (eg, trauma, blood dyscrasia, prematurity)
10. Superior sagittal sinus thrombosis

OBSTRUCTIVE (NONCOMMUNICATING) HYDROCEPHALUS SECONDARY TO INTRAVENTRICULAR, AQUEDUCTAL, FORAMINA OF MONRO, OR FORAMINA OF MAGENDIE AND LUSCHKA OBSTRUCTION

1. Abscess
2. Aneurysm of vein of Galen
3. Arachnoid cyst of suprasellar or quadrigeminal cistern
4. Basal arachnoiditis (incl. tuberculosis, sarcoidosis, fungus disease$_g$)
5. Brain-stem edema
6. Colloid cyst
7. Congenital aqueductal stenosis or occlusion (usually with Arnold-Chiari malformation)
8. Cysticercosis
9. Dandy-Walker S.
10. Hematoma; intraventricular hemorrhage (eg, trauma, AV malformation)
11. Neoplasm, primary (eg, pinealoma, teratoma, craniopharyngioma, intraventricular tumor) or metastatic
12. Tuberous sclerosis

OVERPRODUCTION OF CEREBROSPINAL FLUID

1. Choroid plexus papilloma

References:
1. Brucher JA, Salmon JH: Hydrocephalus. Semin Roentgenol 1970;5:186-195
2. DuBoulay GH (ed): A Textbook of Radiological Diagnosis. (ed 5) The Head and the Central Nervous System. Philadelphia: W.B. Saunders, 1984, vol 1, pp 89-94
3. Eisenberg RL: Clinical Imaging: An Atlas of Differential Diagnosis. (ed 2) Rockville, MD: Aspen Publishers, 1992, pp 860-863

CONGENITAL SYNDROMES ASSOCIATED WITH HYDROCEPHALUS

COMMON

1. Achondroplasia
2. Acrocephalosyndactyly, Apert and Pfeiffer types
3. Arnold-Chiari S.
4. Crouzon S. (craniofacial dysostosis)
5. Dandy-Walker S.
6. Fetal alcohol S.
7. Fetal toxoplasmosis infection
8. Huntington's chorea
9. Mucopolysaccharidosis I-H (Hurler S.) and VI
10 Osteopetrosis, severe

UNCOMMON

1. Acrodysostosis
2. Adrenogenital S.
3. Aminopterin fetopathy
4. Bardet-Biedl S.
5. Basal cell nevus S. (Gorlin)
6. Biemond S. II
7. Cerebrohepatorenal S. (Zellweger S.)
8. Cloverleaf skull
9. Cockayne S.
10. Craniodiaphyseal dysplasia
11. Cystinosis
12. Diencephalic S.
13. Farber disease
14. Incontinentia pigmenti
15. Lissencephaly S.
16. Mannosidosis
17. Meckel S.
18. Metachromatic leukodystrophies
19. Mucopolysaccharidoses I-H (Hurler S.) and VI
20. Oro-facio-digital S. I
21. Osteogenesis imperfecta congenita

22. Rieger S.
23. Riley-Day S.
24. Sjögren-Larsson S.
25. Smith-Lemli-Opitz S.
26. Sotos S.
27. Thanatophoric dysplasia
28. Triploidy S.
29. Trisomy 13 S.
30. Tuberous sclerosis
31. X-linked hydrocephalus

References:

1. Jones KL: Smith's Recognizable Patterns of Human Malformation. Philadelphia: W.B. Saunders, 1988
2. Taybi H, Lachman RS: Radiology of Syndromes, Metabolic
Disorders, and Skeletal Dysplasias. (ed 3) Chicago: Year
Book Medical Publ, 1990, p 861

Subgamut B-48B

LARGE HEADS AND VENTRICLES IN INFANTS

Large Head

WITH LARGE VENTRICLES
1. Hydrocephalus (eg, aqueduct stenosis, Arnold-Chiari
malformation, Dandy-Walker S.)

WITH NORMAL VENTRICLES
1. Calvarial thickening
2. Cerebral edema
3. Intracranial neoplasm or cyst
4. Macrocephaly, megalencephaly (See C-3, C-3A)

Large Ventricles

WITH LARGE HEAD
1. Hydrocephalus (See B-48, B-48A)

WITH NORMAL-SIZED HEAD
1. Cerebral atrophy (eg, intrauterine infection, natal or postnatal anoxia, vascular occlusions)

Reference:
1. Harwood-Nash DCF, Fitz CR: Large heads and ventricles in infants. Radiol Clin North Am 1975;13:199-224

Gamut B-49

LESIONS IDENTIFIABLE ON ULTRASOUND EXAMINATION OF THE INFANT BRAIN

COMMON
1. Hemorrhage involving
   a. Germinal matrix in prematures
   b. Choroid plexus
   c. White matter, in full-term or preterm infant (latter associated with periventricular leucomalacia)
   d. Periventricular or intraventricular in full-term infant
   e. Subdural
2. Hydrocephalus

UNCOMMON
1. Agenesis of corpus callosum
2. Bacterial ventriculitis (occasionally meningitis or encephalitis)
3. Dandy-Walker S.

4. Holoprosencephaly
5. Hydranencephaly, anencephaly
6. Porencephalic cyst (esp. following periventricular hemorrhage)

References:
1. Blomhagen JD, Mack LA: Abnormalities of the neonatal cerebral ventricles. Radiol Clin North Am 1985;23:13-31
2. Chilton SJ, Cremin BJ: Ultrasound diagnosis of CSF cystic lesions in the neonatal brain. Br J Radiol 1983;56:613-620
3. Dewbury K: Ultrasound of the infant brain. In: Grainger RG, Allison DJ (eds): Diagnostic Radiology. Edinburgh: Churchill Livingstone, 1992, vol 3, pp 2089-2095
4. Dewbury KC, Bates RI: Neonatal intracranial hemorrhage: The cause of the ultrasound appearances. Br J Radiol 1983; 56:783-789
5. Mack LA, Rumack CM, Johnson ML: Ultrasound evaluation of cystic intracranial lesions in the neonate. Radiology 1980; 137:451-455

Gamut B-50

CEREBROSPINAL FLUID RHINORRHEA

COMMON
1. Fracture of frontal or sphenoid sinus, or of mastoid sinus
2. Neoplasm of base of skull (esp. osteoma, carcinoma)
3. Postoperative

UNCOMMON
1. Congenital skull defect
2. Hydrocephalus (elevated pressure)
3. Neoplasm of brain or meninges, with erosion
4. Osteomyelitis

Reference:
1. Lantz EJ, Forbes GS, Brown ML, et al: Radiology of cerebrospinal fluid rhinorrhea. AJR 1980;135:1023-1030

CENTRAL NERVOUS SYSTEM COMPLICATIONS OF HIV INFECTION AND AIDS

I. INFECTIONS
1. Bacterial (meningitis or brain abscess)
   a. Tuberculosis
   b. Atypical mycobacterial infection
   c. Syphilis
   d. Other (*E. coli, Listeria, Nocardia*)
2. Fungal$_g$ (meningitis or brain abscess)
   a. Aspergillosis
   b. Candidiasis
   c. Coccidioidomycosis
   d. Cryptococcosis (torulosis)
   e. Histoplasmosis
3. Protozoal
   a. Toxoplasmosis (meningoencephalitis)
4. Viral (encephalopathy, encephalitis)
   a. Human immunodeficiency virus (AIDS)
   b. Cytomegalovirus
   c. Herpes simplex
   d. Herpes zoster
   e. Papovavirus JC (progressive multifocal leuko-encephalopathy - PML)

II. NEOPLASMS
1. Kaposi sarcoma
2. Lymphoma, primary
3. Non-Hodgkin's lymphoma

III. CEREBROVASCULAR DISORDERS
1. Cerebral infarction
2. Intracerebral or subarachnoid hemorrhage

IV. CNS SYNDROMES OF UNCERTAIN ETIOLOGY
1. AIDS-related dementia
2. Aseptic meningitis
3. Vacuolar myelopathy

V. PERIPHERAL NERVOUS SYSTEM DISORDERS
1. Acute polyradiculoneuropathy (eg, Guillian-Barré S.)
2. Chronic inflammatory demyelinating polyneuropathy
3. Distal symmetrical axonal polyneuropathy
4. Mononeuritis multiplex

References:
1. Eisenberg RL: Clinical Imaging: An Atlas of Differential Diagnosis. (ed 2) Rockville, MD: Aspen Publishers, 1992, pp 958-961
2. Moseley IF, Murray JF, Goodman PC: HIV infection and AIDS: Central nervous system complications. In: Grainger RG, Allison DJ (eds): Diagnostic Radiology. Edinburgh: Churchill Livingstone, 1992, vol 3, pp 1994-1997

C

Calvarium (Skull)

ABNORMAL SIZE OR SHAPE

ABNORMAL DENSITY OR THICKNESS

DESTRUCTION

SELLA TURCICA

BASE OF SKULL

MISCELLANEOUS

C

Gamut C-1

PREMATURE CRANIOSYNOSTOSIS (CRANIOSTENOSIS)

COMMON
1. Congenital syndromes (See C-1B)
*2. Decreased intracranial pressure (brain atrophy, shunted hydrocephalus - "contracting skull")
3. Primary (idiopathic) craniosynostosis (See C-1A)

UNCOMMON
*1. Anemia$_g$ (eg, sickle cell, thalassemia, iron deficiency)
*2. Cretinism, hypothyroidism (treated)
*3. Hyperthyroidism
*4. Hypervitaminosis D
5. Microcephaly (failure of brain growth)
*6. Polycythemia vera
*7. Rickets (hypophosphatemic, treated; vitamin D resistant)

*Secondary synostosis.

References:
1. Cohen MM Jr: Genetic perspective on craniosynostosis and syndromes with craniosynostosis. Neurosurgery 1977;47: 886
2. David DJ, Poswillo D, Simpson D: The Craniosynostoses. Berlin: Springer-Verlag, 1982
3. Duggan CA, Keever EB, Gay BB Jr: Secondary craniosynostosis. AJR 1970;109:277-293
4. Jones KL: Smith's Recognizable Patterns of Human Malformation. (ed 3) Philadelphia: W.B. Saunders, 1988
5. Newton TH, Potts DG: Radiology of the Skull and Brain. St. Louis: C.V. Mosby, 1971, vol 1, book 1, pp 222-228
6. Swischuk LE: Differential Diagnosis in Pediatric Radiology. Baltimore: Williams & Wilkins, 1984, p 350
7. Taybi H, Lachman RS: Radiology of Syndromes, Metabolic Disorders, and Skeletal Dysplasias. (ed 3) Chicago: Year Book Medical Publ, 1990, p 852

Subgamut C-1A

CLASSIFICATION OF PRIMARY (IDIOPATHIC) PREMATURE CRANIOSYNOSTOSIS

1. Brachycephaly (short, wide, slightly high head with "harlequin" orbits) - bilateral coronal sutures
2. Microcephaly (small round head) - all sutures (universal craniosynostosis)
3. Oxycephaly (tall, wide, short head) or turricephaly (tower-shaped, pointed head with overgrowth of bregma and flat, underdeveloped lower posterior fossa) - bilateral lambdoid and coronal sutures
4. Plagiocephaly (oblique asymmetrical head) - unilateral coronal suture (with flattening of ipsilateral frontoparietal region, elevation of ipsilateral sphenoid wing, and unilateral "harlequin" orbit) and/or lambdoid suture
5. Scaphocephaly (boat head) or dolichocephaly (long, narrow, slightly high head) - sagittal suture
6. Trigonocephaly (triangular head; narrow in front, broad behind with hypotelorism) - metopic suture
7. Triphyllocephaly (cloverleaf skull or kleeblattschädel) - trilobular skull with frontal and temporal bulges - intrauterine premature closure of sagittal, coronal, and lambdoid sutures

References:
1. Newton TH, Potts DG: Radiology of the Skull and Brain. St. Louis: C.V. Mosby, 1971, vol 1, book 1, p 222
2. Silverman FN (ed): Caffey's Pediatric X-ray Diagnosis. (ed 8) Chicago: Year Book Medical Publ, 1985, pp 36-43
3. Swischuk LE: Differential Diagnosis in Pediatric Radiology. Baltimore: Williams & Wilkins, 1984, p 331
4. Swischuk LE: Imaging of the Newborn, Infant, and Young Child. (ed 3) Baltimore: Williams & Wilkins, 1989, pp 906-913

Subgamut C-1B

CONGENITAL SYNDROMES WITH PREMATURE CRANIOSYNOSTOSIS

COMMON

1. Achondroplasia (base of skull)
2. Acrocephalopolysyndactyly (Carpenter and other types)
3. Acrocephalosyndactyly (Apert and other types)
4. Asphyxiating thoracic dysplasia
5. Chondrodysplasia punctata (Conradi's disease)
6. Cloverleaf skull (kleeblattschädel)
7. Craniofacial dysostosis (Crouzon S.)
8. Hypophosphatasia (late)
9. Mucopolysaccharidoses (eg, Hurler S.; Maroteaux-Lamy S.); mucolipidosis III; fucosidosis
10. Rubella S.
11. Thanatophoric dysplasia
12. Trisomy 21 S. (Down S.)

UNCOMMON

1. Acrocraniofacial dysostosis
2. Adducted thumb S. (Christian S.)
3. Adrenogenital S.
4. Aminopterin fetopathy
5. Baller-Gerold S.
6. Bird-headed dwarfism (Seckel S.)
7. C S.
8. Chromosomal syndromes (5p-, 7q+, 13)
9. Craniotelencephalic dysplasia
10. Fetal hydantoin S.
11. Fetal trimethadione S.
12. Idiopathic hypercalcemia (Williams S.)
13. Meckel S.
14. Metaphyseal chondrodysplasia (Jansen)
15. Oculo-mandibulo-facial S. (Hallermann-Streiff S.)
16. Osteoglophonic dysplasia
17. Trisomy 18 S.

References:
1. Cohen MM Jr: Genetic perspective on craniosynostosis and syndromes with craniosynostosis. Neurosurgery 1977;47: 886
2. David DJ, Poswillo D, Simpson D: The Craniosynostoses. Berlin: Springer-Verlag, 1982
3. Jones KL: Smith's Recognizable Patterns of Human Malformation. Philadelphia:W.B. Saunders, 1988
4. Newton TH, Potts DG: Radiology of the Skull and Brain. St. Louis: C.V. Mosby, 1971, vol 1, book 1, pp 222-228
5. Swischuk LE: Differential Diagnosis in Pediatric Radiology. Baltimore:Williams & Wilkins, 1984, p 350
6. Taybi H, Lachman RS: Radiology of Syndromes, Metabolic Disorders, and Skeletal Dysplasias. (ed 3) Chicago:Year Book Medical Publ, 1990, p 852

Gamut C-2

MICROCEPHALY (MICROCRANIA)

COMMON
1. Cerebral atrophy; perinatal brain damage from hypoxia
2. Craniosynostosis, total
3. Encephalocele
4. Idiopathic small brain (micrencephaly)
5. Prenatal irradiation or infection (eg, toxoplasmosis, rubella, cytomegalovirus, herpes, syphilis)

UNCOMMON
1. Adducted thumb S.
2. Aminopterin fetopathy
3. Beckwith-Wiedemann S.
4. Bird-headed dwarfism (Seckel S.)
5. C S.
6. Cephaloskeletal dysplasia (Taybi-Linder S.)
7. Cerebro-oculo-facial-skeletal S.
8. Chondrodysplasia punctata (Conradi's disease)
9. Chromosome syndromes [eg, 4p-, 5p-(cat cry S.), 18q-,22]
10. Cockayne S.
11. Coffin-Siris S.

12. Cornelia de Lange S.
13. Deprivation dwarfism
14. Dubowitz S.
15. Dyggve-Melchior-Clausen S.
16. Familial
17. Fanconi anemia
18. Fetal alcohol S.
19. Fetal hydantoin S.
20. Fetal trimethadione S.
21. Goltz S.
22. "Happy puppet" S.
23. Holoprosencephaly (arhinencephaly)
24. Homocystinuria
25. Incontinentia pigmenti
26. Johanson-Blizzard S.
27. Kinky-hair S. (Menkes S.)
28. Langer-Giedion S.
29. Lenz microphthalmia S.
30. Lesch-Nyhan S.
31. Lissencephaly S.
32. Meckel S.
33. Noonan S.
34. [Normal variant]
35. Prader-Willi S.
36. Riley-Day S.
37. Rubinstein-Taybi S.
38. Smith-Lemli-Opitz S.
39. Trisomy 13 S.
40. Trisomy 18 S.
41. Trisomy 21 S. (Down S.)

References:

1. Felson B (ed): Dwarfs and other little people. Semin Roentgenol 1973:8:133-263
2. Newton TH, Potts DG: Radiology of the Skull and Brain. St. Louis: C.V. Mosby, 1971, vol 1, book 1, pp 151-152
3. Jones KL: Smith's Recognizable Patterns of Human Malformation. Philadelphia: W.B. Saunders, 1988
4. Taybi H, Lachman RS: Radiology of Syndromes, Metabolic Disorders, and Skeletal Dysplasias. (ed 3) Chicago: Year Book Medical Publ, 1990, p 854

Gamut C-3

MACROCEPHALY (MACROCRANIA)

COMMON
1. [Calvarial thickening (eg, congenital anemias$_g$)]
*2. Congenital syndromes (See C-3A)
*3. Craniostenosis
4. Hydrocephalus (See B-48, B-48A)
*5. Subdural hematoma

UNCOMMON
1. Aneurysm of vein of Galen
2. Aqueduct stenosis
3. Arnold-Chiari malformation
4. Choroid plexus papilloma
*5. Expansion of middle fossa (See C-27)
6. Hydranencephaly
7. Infection causing hydrocephalus (eg, meningitis, toxoplasmosis)
8. Megalencephaly
9. Porencephaly
10. Posterior fossa cyst (eg, dermoid, teratoma, Dandy-Walker S.)
*11. Tumor or subarachnoid cyst adjacent to calvarium

*May be asymmetrical.

References:

1. Harwood-Nash DC, Fitz CR: Large heads and ventricles in infants. Radiol Clin North Am 1975;13:119-224
2. Newton TH, Potts DG: Radiology of the Skull and Brain. St. Louis: C.V. Mosby, 1971, vol 1, book 1, pp 144-151
3. Scotti LN, Maravilla K, Hardman DR: The enlarging head - angiographic evaluation of megacephaly. American Roentgen Ray Society Scientific Exhibit, Atlanta, 1975
4. Swischuk LE: Differential Diagnosis in Pediatric Radiology. Baltimore: Williams & Wilkins, 1984, pp 329-330

Subgamut C-3A

CONGENITAL SYNDROMES WITH MACROCEPHALY*

COMMON

1. Achondroplasia, hypochondroplasia
2. Hydrocephalus (See B-48A)
3. Hyperostosis diseases (eg, osteopetrosis, craniometaphyseal dysplasia, Camurati-Engelmann disease, pyknodysostosis, hyperphosphatasia)
4. Mucopolysaccharides$_g$ (incl. Hurler, Hunter, Morquio, Maroteaux-Lamy); GM$_1$ gangliosidosis
5. Neurofibromatosis

UNCOMMON

1. Achondrogenesis, hypochondrogenesis
2. Beckwith-Wiedemann S.
3. Campomelic dysplasia
4. Cerebral gigantism (Sotos S.)
5. Cerebrohepatorenal S. (Zellweger S.)
6. Cleidocranial dysplasia
7. Cranioectodermal dysplasia
8. Dandy-Walker S.
9. Familial megalencephaly; megalencephaly syndromes
10. Greig cephalopolysyndactyly S.
11. Hypomelanosis of Ito
12. Klippel-Trenaunay-Weber S.
13. Kniest dysplasia
14. Marfan S.
15. Noonan S.
16. Osteogenesis imperfecta
17. Pituitary gigantism or dwarfism
18. Proteus S.
19. Riley-Smith S.
20. Robinow S.
21. Schwarz-Lélek S.
22. [Silver-Russell S.]
23. Spondyloepiphyseal dysplasia congenita (lethal)

24. Tay-Sachs disease
25. Thanatophoric dysplasia
26. Tuberous sclerosis

* Many dwarfs have relative macrocephaly.

References:

1. DeMyer W: Megalencephaly in children: clinical syndromes, genetic patterns, and differential diagnoses from other causes of megalocephaly. Neurology 1972;22:634-643
2. Holt JF, Kuhns LR: Macrocranium and macrocephaly in neurofibromatosis. Skeletal Radiol 1976;1:25-28
3. Jones KL: Smith's Recognizable Patterns of Human Malformation. Philadelphia: W.B. Saunders, 1988
4. Swischuk LE: Differential Diagnosis in Pediatric Radiology. Baltimore: Williams & Wilkins, 1984, p 329
5. Taybi H, Lachman RS: Radiology of Syndromes, Metabolic Disorders, and Skeletal Dysplasias. (ed 3) Chicago: Year Book Medical Publ, 1990, pp 853-854

Gamut C-4

ABNORMAL CONTOUR OF THE CALVARIUM
(See Gamuts C-1 to C-11)

COMMON

1. Achondroplasia, other congenital syndromes (See C-1 to C-11)
2. Fibrous dysplasia, leontiasis ossea
3. Hemiatrophy of brain (eg, Sturge-Weber S.; Dyke-Davidoff-Masson S.); localized cerebral atrophy
4. Hydrocephalus
5. Paget's disease (eg, tam-o'-shanter skull) (See C-4A)
6. Postoperative
7. Postural flattening, usually occipital (eg, cerebral palsy); postural asymmetry from scoliosis
8. Premature craniosynostosis (See C-1, C-1A)
9. Trauma (incl. obstetrical)

UNCOMMON
1. Arachnoid cyst
2. Craniolacunia
3. Craniofacial dysostosis (Crouzon S.)
4. Craniopagus twins
5. Dandy-Walker S.
6. Encephalocele
7. Hyperphosphatasia
8. Hypertelorism (See H-3); cranium bifidum
9. Microcephaly
10. Neoplasm
11. Neurofibromatosis
12. Porencephalic cyst; cerebral cyst
13. Rickets, healed, with bossing
14. Silver-Russell S.
15. Subdural hematoma, chronic; hygroma

Subgamut C-4A

TAM-O'-SHANTER SKULL (THICKENING OF THE SKULL VAULT WITH BASILAR INVAGINATION)

COMMON
1. Paget's disease

UNCOMMON
1. Fibrous dysplasia
2. Hypophosphatasia
3. Neurofibromatosis
4. Osteogenesis imperfecta
5. Osteomalacia, rickets

Gamut C-5

UNILATERAL SMALL CRANIUM

COMMON
1. Cerebral hemiatrophy (eg, Dyke-Davidoff-Masson S.; Sturge-Weber S.)
2. Normal (slight)
3. Trauma (depressed skull fracture)
4. Unilateral lambdoid or coronal craniosynostosis

UNCOMMON
1. Head positioning in infancy (postural flattening)
2. Radiation therapy
3. Silver-Russell S. (congenital hemiatrophy)

Gamut C-6

ABNORMAL CONTOUR OF THE OCCIPUT (FLAT OR PROMINENT) IN AN INFANT

Flat

COMMON
1. Achondroplasia
2. Postural flattening (eg, normal, mentally retarded, or immobilized infant)
3. Trisomy 21 S. (Down S.)

UNCOMMON
1. Acrocephalopolysyndactyly (Carpenter S.)
2. Acrocephalosyndactyly (Apert S.)
3. Craniofacial dysostosis (Crouzon S.)
4. Mucopolysaccharidosis III (Sanfilippo S.)
5. XXXXY S.

Prominent

COMMON
1. Bathrocephaly (idiopathic)
2. Dandy-Walker S.; posterior fossa arachnoid cyst

UNCOMMON
1. Cephalhematoma, occipital
2. Engelmann's disease
3. Hajdu-Cheney S. (idiopathic osteolysis)
4. Meningocele, occipital
5. Otopalatodigital S.
6. Pyknodysostosis
7. Trisomy 18 S.

Reference:
1. Jones KL: Smith's Recognizable Patterns of Human Malformation. (ed 3) Philadelphia: W.B. Saunders, 1988

Gamut C-7

FRONTAL BOSSING
(PROMINENT CENTRAL FOREHEAD)

COMMON
1. Achondroplasia
2. Anemia$_g$ (esp. sickle cell, thalassemia)
3. Rickets, healed

UNCOMMON
1. Achondrogenesis
2. Basal cell nevus S. (Gorlin S.)
3. Cleidocranial dysplasia
4. Cranio-fronto-nasal dysplasia
5. Craniometaphyseal dysplasia
6. Craniotelencephalic dysplasia

7. Diastrophic dysplasia
8. Engelmann's disease (diaphyseal dysplasia)
9. Frontometaphyseal dysplasia
10. Goldenhar-Gorlin S.
11. Greig cephalopolysyndactyly S.
12. Hydrocephalus
13. Hypochondroplasia
14. Larsen S.
15. Lissencephaly S.
16. Lowe S.
17. Marshall-Smith S.
18. Megalencephaly
19. Metatropic dysplasia
20. Mucopolysaccharidoses (Hurler S.); mucolipidosis II; GM_1 gangliosidosis
21. Oculo-mandibulo-facial S. (Hallermann-Streiff S.)
22. Oro-facio-digital S. I (Papillon-Leage S.)
23. Osteoglophonic dysplasia
24. Osteopetrosis, severe
25. Otopalatodigital S.
26. Progeria
27. Pyknodysostosis
28. Riley-Smith S.
29. Robinow S.
30. Schwarz-Lélek S.
31. Sclerosteosis
32. Silver-Russell S.
33. Sotos S.
34. Subdural hematoma, chronic
35. Thanatophoric dysplasia
36. 3-M S.
37. Trisomy 8 S.

References:
1. Jones KL: Smith's Recognizable Patterns of Human Malformation. (ed 3) Philadelphia: W.B. Saunders, 1988
2. Swischuk LE: Differential Diagnosis in Pediatric Radiology. Baltimore: Williams & Wilkins, 1984, p 335
3. Taybi H, Lachman RS: Radiology of Syndromes, Metabolic Disorders, and Skeletal Dysplasias. (ed 3) Chicago: Year Book Medical Publ, 1990, p 853

Gamut C-8

BIPARIETAL BOSSING

1. Bilateral coronal synostosis, isolated or with Crouzon S.
2. Bilateral subdural hematoma, chronic
3. Cleidocranial dysplasia
4. Cloverleaf skull (kleeblattschädel)
5. Pyknodysostosis
6. Rickets, healed

Reference:
1. Swischuk LE: Differential Diagnosis in Pediatric Radiology. Baltimore: Williams & Wilkins, 1984, p 336

Gamut C-9

LOCALIZED BULGE OF THE CALVARIUM OR SCALP

COMMON
1. Anemia, chronic$_g$ (eg, sickle cell, iron deficiency)
2. Cephalhematoma
3. Metastatic carcinoma or neuroblastoma
4. Myeloma

UNCOMMON
1. Arachnoid cyst with erosion
2. Dermoid cyst, intradiploic
3. Fibrous dysplasia
4. Histiocytosis X$_g$
5. Intracranial neoplasm (large) with erosion of calvarium
6. Leptomeningeal cyst
7. Meningioma
8. Paget's disease with secondary malignant neoplasm
9. Porencephalic cyst

10. Primary neoplasm of calvarium (eg, sarcoma, osteoma)
11. Scalp neoplasm or cyst
12. Subdural hematoma

Reference:
1. Swischuk LE: Differential Diagnosis in Pediatric Radiology. Baltimore: Williams & Wilkins, 1984, p 337

Gamut C-10

BASILAR INVAGINATION

COMMON
1. Arnold-Chiari malformation
2. Congenital craniovertebral anomaly (See S-10)
   a. Atlantoaxial dislocation with or without congenital separation of odontoid
   b. Atlanto-occipital fusion (assimilation)
   c. Klippel-Feil S.
   d. Stenosis of foramen magnum
   e. Unfused posterior arch of atlas
3. Osteogenesis imperfecta
4. Osteomalacia; rickets
5. Paget's disease

UNCOMMON
1. Achondroplasia
2. Aqueduct stenosis
3. Cleidocranial dysplasia
4. Craniofacial dysostosis (Crouzon S.)
5. Fibrous dysplasia
6. Hajdu-Cheney S. (idiopathic acro-osteolysis)
7. Histiocytosis X_g
8. Hydrocephalus, chronic
9. Hyperparathyroidism, primary or secondary (renal osteodystrophy)

10. Hypophosphatasia
11. Mucopolysaccharidoses (eg, Hurler, Morquio)
12. Occipital craniotomy in a child
13. Osteomyelitis (incl. syphilis, tuberculosis)
14. Osteopetrosis
15. Osteoporosis
16. Psoriatic arthritis
17. Pyknodysostosis
18. Rheumatoid arthritis; ankylosing spondylitis
19. Trauma, severe
20. Trisomy 21 S. (Down S.)

References:
1. Dolan KD: Cervicobasilar relationships. Radiol Clin North Am 1977;15:155-166
2. DuBoulay GH: Principles of X-ray Diagnosis of the Skull. (ed 2) London: Butterworths, 1980, pp 229-235
3. Epstein BS, Epstein JA: The association of cerebellar tonsillar herniation with basilar impression incident to Paget's disease. AJR 1969;107:535-542
4. Taybi H, Lachman RS: Radiology of Syndromes, Metabolic Disorders, and Skeletal Dysplasias. (ed 3) Chicago: Year Book Medical Publ, 1990, pp 851-852

Gamut C-11

HYPOPLASIA OF THE BASE OF THE SKULL

COMMON
1. Achondroplasia
2. Cretinism
3. Trisomy 21 S. (Down S.)

UNCOMMON
1. Achondrogenesis
2. Acrocephalopolysyndactyly (Carpenter S.)
3. Acrocephalosyndactyly (Apert, Pfeiffer types)
4. Cranial dysplasia; cleidocranial dysplasia

5. Craniofacial dysostosis (Crouzon S.)
6. Oculo-mandibulo-facial S. (Hallermann-Streiff S.)
7. Orbital hypotelorism with arhinencephaly; trisomy 13 S.
8. Short rib-polydactyly S.
9. Thanatophoric dysplasia

References:
1. Dorst J: Personal communication
2. DuBoulay GH: Principles of X-ray Diagnosis of the Skull. (ed 2) London: Butterworths, 1980, pp 237-243

Gamut C-12

LOCALIZED INCREASED DENSITY, SCLEROSIS, OR THICKENING OF THE CALVARIUM

COMMON
1. Anatomic variation (eg, sutural sclerosis; external occipital protuberance)
2. Anemia$_g$ (esp. sickle cell)
3. [Artifact; hair braid; overlying soft tissue tumor or sebaceous cyst]
4. Cephalhematoma; ossified subdural hematoma
5. Chronic osteomyelitis or adjacent cellulitis; tuberculosis; syphilis; mycetoma
6. [Depressed skull fracture]
7. Fibrous dysplasia
8. Hyperostosis frontalis interna
*9. Meningioma
*10. Metastasis, osteoblastic (eg, prostate, breast)
11. Osteoma
12. Paget's disease

UNCOMMON
1. Arteriovenous malformation of dura
2. Cerebral hemiatrophy; Davidoff-Dyke S.
3. [Dural calcification]

C. Calvarium (Skull)

4. Frontometaphyseal dysplasia
*5. Hemangioma
6. Histiocytosis X_g, healing
7. Ischemic necrosis (eg, bone flap)
8. Lymphoma$_g$
9. Mastocytosis
10. Neurofibromatosis
11. Osteoblastoma
12. Osteochondroma
*13. Osteosarcoma
14. Radiation osteonecrosis; treated tumor (eg, brown tumor, lytic metastasis from breast)
15. Tuberous sclerosis

* Sunburst spiculations may be present.

Reference:

1. DuBoulay GH: Principles of X-ray Diagnosis of the Skull. (ed 2) London: Butterworths, 1980, pp 113-125

Gamut C-13

DIFFUSE OR WIDESPREAD INCREASED DENSITY, SCLEROSIS, OR THICKENING OF THE CALVARIUM

COMMON

1. Acromegaly
*2. Anemia$_g$ (sickle cell, thalassemia, iron deficiency, hereditary spherocytosis)
3. Cerebral atrophy in childhood (contracting skull)
4. Congenital syndromes; sclerosing bone dysplasias (See C-13A)
+5. Fibrous dysplasia, leontiasis ossea
6. Hydrocephalus, postshunting
7. Hyperostosis interna generalisata; Morgagni-Stewart-Morel S.

8. Hyperparathyroidism, primary or secondary, treated (renal osteodystrophy, esp. in patients on dialysis)
9. Normal, idiopathic
*10. Metastases, osteoblastic (eg, prostate, breast)
11. Myelosclerosis
12. Paget's disease ("cotton wool" appearance)

UNCOMMON

1. AV malformation, large
2. Craniosynostosis (See C-1)
3. Cretinism, hypothyroidism (treated)
4. Cyanotic congenital heart disease, long standing
5. Dilantin therapy (chronic)
6. Dystrophia myotonica
7. Fluorosis
8. Hemihypertrophy of cranium due to cerebral hemiatrophy (Dyke-Davidoff-Masson S.)
9. Homocystinuria
10. Hypervitaminosis D
11. Hypoparathyroidism
12. Increased intracranial pressure in adults, chronic (eg, from intermittent obstruction)
13. Infantile cortical hyperostosis (Caffey's disease)
*14. Leukemia, lymphoma$_g$
*15. Meningioma
16. Microcephaly
*17. Neuroblastoma metastases
18. Osteomyelitis, chronic; mycetoma
*19. Polycythemia (childhood)
20. Rickets, treated ("bossing"); vitamin D-resistant rickets
21. Syphilitic osteitis

* May show vertical striations ("hair on end").
\+ May develop leontiasis ossea (lion-like facies) due to overgrowth of facial bones.

References:

1. Anderson R, et al: Thickening of the skull in surgically treated hydrocephalus. AJR 1970;110:96-101
2. DuBoulay GH: Principles of X-ray Diagnosis of the Skull. (ed 2) London: Butterworths, 1980, pp 98-113

3. Griscom NT, Oh KS: The contracting skull; Inward growth of the inner table as a physiologic response to diminution of intracranial content in children. AJR 1970;110:106-110

4. Kattan KR: Calvarial thickening after Dilantin medication. AJR 1970;110:102-105

5. Swischuk LE: Differential Diagnosis in Pediatric Radiology. Baltimore: Williams & Wilkins, 1984, pp 338-341

6. Taybi H, Lachman RS: Radiology of Syndromes, Metabolic Disorders, and Skeletal Dysplasias. (ed 3) Chicago: Year Book Medical Publ, 1990

7. Teplick JG, Haskin ME: Roentgenologic Diagnosis. (ed 3) Philadelphia: W.B. Saunders, 1976

Subgamut C-13A

CONGENITAL CONDITIONS WITH INCREASED DENSITY OR THICKENING OF THE CALVARIUM

COMMON

+1. Craniometaphyseal dysplasia; metaphyseal dysplasia (Pyle's disease); frontometaphyseal dysplasia

2. Craniosynostosis (See C-1)

3. Cretinism, hypothyroidism

4. Cyanotic congenital heart disease, long standing

5. Endosteal hyperostosis (van Buchem S., Worth S.)

6. Engelmann's disease (diaphyseal dysplasia)

7. Fanconi anemia

+8. Fibrous dysplasia (leontiasis ossea) (incl. McCune-Albright S.)

9. Hemihypertrophy of cranium due to cerebral hemitrophy (Dyke-Davidoff-Masson S.)

10. Homocystinuria

+11. Hyperphosphatasia

12. Microcephaly

13. Mucopolysaccharidoses; GM_1 gangliosidosis

14. Osteopetrosis

15. Pachydermoperiostosis

16. Pseudohypoparathyroidism;
    pseudopseudohypoparathyroidism
17. Pyknodysostosis
18. Tuberous sclerosis

UNCOMMON

1. Acrodysostosis
2. Adrenogenital S.
3. Cockayne S.
4. Craniodiaphyseal dysplasia
5. Distal osteosclerosis
6. Dysosteosclerosis
7. Idiopathic hypercalcemia (Williams S.)
8. Lawrence-Seip S.
9. Lenz-Majewski hyperostotic dwarfism
10. Marshall S.
11. Melorheostosis
12. Oculo-dento-osseous dysplasia
13. Osteodysplasty (Melnick-Needles S.)
14. Osteogenesis imperfecta tarda
15. Osteopathia striata
16. Otopalatodigital S.
17. Schwarz-Lélek S.
18. Sclerosteosis
19. Troell-Junet S.
20. Tubular stenosis (Kenny-Caffey S.)
21. Weill-Marchesani S.
22. XXXXY S.

+ May develop leontiasis ossea (lion-like facies) due to overgrowth of facial bones.

References:

1. Kozlowski K., Beighton P.: Gamut Index of Skeletal Dysplasias. Berlin: Springer-Verlag, 1984
2. Swischuk LE: Differential Diagnosis in Pediatric Radiology. Baltimore: Williams & Wilkins, 1984, pp 338-341
3. Taybi H, Lachman RS: Radiology of Syndromes, Metabolic Disorders, and Skeletal Dysplasias. (ed 3) Chicago: Year Book Medical Publ, 1990

Gamut C-14

LOCALIZED INCREASED DENSITY, SCLEROSIS, OR THICKENING OF THE BASE OF THE SKULL
(See Gamut C-15)

COMMON
1. Fibrous dysplasia
2. Mastoiditis, chronic sclerotic
3. Meningioma

UNCOMMON
1. Chordoma (with calcification)
2. Lymphoepithelioma of nasopharynx or paranasal sinus
3. Lymphoma$_g$
4. Metastasis, osteoblastic
5. Nasopharyngeal infection, chronic (eg, tuberculosis)
6. Osteoma; chondroma
7. Petrositis or osteomyelitis, chronic
8. Radiation therapy for invasive carcinoma of ear, sphenoid sinus, or nasopharynx
9. Sarcoma (eg, osteosarcoma, chondrosarcoma, rhabdomyosarcoma)
10. Sphenoid sinusitis; mucocele

References:
1. Potter GD: Sclerosis of the base of the skull as a manifestation of nasopharyngeal carcinoma. Radiology 1970;94:35-38
2. Tsai FY, Lisella RS, Lee KF, et al: Osteosclerosis of base of skull as a manifestation of tumor invasion. AJR 1975;124: 256-264

Gamut C-15

GENERALIZED INCREASED DENSITY, SCLEROSIS, OR THICKENING OF THE BASE OF THE SKULL
(See Gamut C-14)

COMMON
1. Fibrous dysplasia
2. Paget's disease

UNCOMMON
1. Anemia$_g$, primary (eg, thalassemia, sickle cell)
2. Cleidocranial dysplasia
3. Craniometaphyseal dysplasia
4. Cretinism
5. Engelmann's disease (diaphyseal dysplasia)
6. Fluorosis
7. Frontometaphyseal dysplasia
8. Hyperparathyroidism, primary or secondary (treated)
9. Hypervitaminosis D
10. Idiopathic hypercalcemia (Williams S.)
11. Melorheostosis
12. Meningioma
13. Metaphyseal chondrodysplasia (Jansen)
14. Metaphyseal dysplasia (Pyle's disease)
15. Neurofibromatosis
16. Osteodysplasty (Melnick-Needles S.)
17. Osteopathia striata
18. Osteopetrosis
19. Otopalatodigital S.
20. Pachydermoperiostosis
21. Pyknodysostosis
22. Ribbing's disease (hereditary multiple diaphyseal sclerosis)
23. Tricho-dento-osseous S.
24. Vitamin D-resistant rickets (healing)

References:
1. DuBoulay GH: Principles of X-ray Diagnosis of the Skull. (ed 2) London: Butterworths, 1980
2. Swischuk LE: Differential Diagnosis in Pediatric Radiology. Baltimore: Williams & Wilkins, 1984, p 344

Gamut C-16

THINNING OF THE SKULL, LOCALIZED OR GENERALIZED

Localized

COMMON
1. Parietal thinning
2. Subdural hematoma, chronic

UNCOMMON
1. Congenital arachnoid cyst
2. Intracranial tumor, slow growing
3. Leptomeningeal cyst
4. Localized cerebral agenesis or atrophy
5. Localized temporal horn hydrocephalus
6. Necrosis of skull (eg, radiation therapy)
7. Neurofibromatosis
8. Porencephalic cyst

Generalized

COMMON
1. Craniolacunia
2. Hydrocephalus, long standing
3. Normal (eg, prematurity)
4. Osteogenesis imperfecta

UNCOMMON

1. Aminopterin fetopathy
2. Cleidocranial dysplasia; cranial dysplasia
3. Hypophosphatasia
4. Increased intracranial pressure, other causes (See B-47)
5. Osteodysplasty (Melnick-Needles S.)
6. Progeria
7. Rickets
8. Trisomy 18 S.

References:

1. DuBoulay GH: Principles of X-ray Diagnosis of the Skull. (ed 2) London: Butterworths, 1980
2. Swischuk LE: Differential Diagnosis in Pediatric Radiology. Baltimore: Williams & Wilkins, 1984, pp 346-347

Gamut C-17

DIFFUSE OR WIDESPREAD DEMINERALIZATION OR DESTRUCTION OF THE SKULL (INCLUDING "SALT AND PEPPER" SKULL)

COMMON

*1. Hyperparathyroidism, primary or secondary
*2. Leukemia, lymphoma$_g$
*3. Metastatic carcinoma or neuroblastoma
*4. Multiple myeloma
*5. Osteomyelitis, diffuse
 6. Osteoporosis (eg, senile, postmenopausal)

UNCOMMON

1. Anemia$_g$ (eg, sickle cell, thalassemia)
2. Electric burn; thermal burn
3. Idiopathic

4. Meningioma or other meningeal neoplasm
5. Osteomalacia; rickets
6. Osteonecrosis
*7. Paget's disease (osteoporosis circumscripta)
8. Primary malignant neoplasm of skull (eg, Ewing's sarcoma)
9. Radiation necrosis; radium poisoning
10. Steroid therapy; Cushing S.
11. Syphilis

* May show mottled or "salt and pepper" destruction of calvarium.

Gamut C-18

EROSION OF THE INNER TABLE OF THE SKULL

COMMON
1. Metastasis
2. Osteomyelitis
3. Pacchionian granulation
4. Subdural hematoma, chronic

UNCOMMON
1. AV malformation of brain surface
2. Cisterna magna anomaly
3. Epidermoid
4. Glioma or cyst of superficial brain cortex (eg, oligodendroglioma, leptomeningeal cyst)
5. Hemangioma of skull
6. Histiocytosis X_g (esp. eosinophilic granuloma)
7. Meningioma
8. Multiple myeloma
9. Neoplasm of dura, other (eg, sarcoma, melanoma)
10. Porencephaly
11. Sinus pericranii

Gamut C-19

BUTTON SEQUESTRUM OF THE SKULL*

COMMON
1. Eosinophilic granuloma
2. Metastatic carcinoma (esp. breast)
3. Osteomyelitis

UNCOMMON
1. [Burr hole or bone flap]
2. [Calvarial "doughnut", idiopathic]
3. Dermoid cyst
4. Epidermoid (primary cholesteatoma)
5. Fibrosing osteitis
6. [Hemangioma]
7. Meningioma
8. Multiple myeloma
9. Necrosis (eg, radiation therapy, radium poisoning, electric burn, electric shock therapy)
10. Paget's disease
11. Sarcoidosis
12. Syphilis
13. Tuberculosis

* Round radiolucent skull defect with central bony density or sequestrum.

References:
1. Newton TH, Potts DG: Radiology of the Skull and Brain. St. Louis: C.V. Mosby, 1971, p 759
2. Rosen IW, Nadel HI: Button sequestrum of the skull. Radiology 1969;92:969-971
3. Satin R, Usher MS, Goldenberg M: More causes of button sequestrum. J Can Assoc Radiol 1976;27:288-289
4. Sholkoff SD, Mainzer F: Button sequestrum revisited. Radiology 1971;100:649-652
5. Wells PO: Button sequestrum of eosinophilic granuloma of the skull. Radiology 1956;67:746-747

Gamut C-20

SOLITARY OSTEOLYTIC SKULL LESION
(See Gamut C-21)

COMMON
*1. Cholesteatoma (inflammatory)
*2. Epidermoid (primary cholesteatoma)
*3. Fibrous dysplasia
 4. Fracture (esp. depressed)
*5. Hemangioma
*6. Histiocytosis X_g (esp. eosinophilic granuloma)
*7. Meningocele, encephalocele, cranium bifidum
 8. Metastasis
 9. Myeloma, plasmacytoma
10. Normal variant (eg, venous lake, enlarged emissary channel, inioindineal canal, pacchionian granulation, parietal foramen, parietal thinning) (See C-35)
*11. Osteomyelitis
12. Paget's disease (osteoporosis circumscripta)
*13. Surgical defect (eg, burr hole, craniotomy flap)

UNCOMMON
 1. Arachnoid cyst
 2. AV malformation
 3. Brown tumor of hyperparathyroidism
*4. Calvarial "doughnut", idiopathic
 5. Dermal sinus
 6. Dermoid cyst
 7. Ectopic glial tissue (occipital)
 8. Fibrosing osteitis
 9. Glomus jugulare tumor (base)
10. Hydatid cyst
11. Idiopathic
12. Intraosseous or chronic subdural hematoma
13. Leptomeningeal cyst
*14. Lymphoma$_g$
*15. Mucocele or neoplasm of paranasal sinus
*16. Necrosis of skull (eg, radiation therapy, electrical or thermal burn)

*17. Neoplasm of brain or dura with bone erosion (esp. meningioma)
18. Neoplasm or cyst of scalp (eg, carcinoma, rodent ulcer, neurofibroma, sebaceous cyst)
19. Neoplasm of skull, benign
20. Neurofibromatosis (eg, asterion or lambdoid suture defect, absent sphenoid wing)
*21. Sarcoidosis
22. Sarcoma of bone
*23. Syphilis
*24. Tuberculosis, fungus disease$_g$

* May have surrounding sclerosis.

References:
1. DuBoulay GH; Principles of X-ray Diagnosis of the Skull. (ed 2) London: Butterworths, 1980, pp 57-94
2. Lane B: Erosions of the skull. Radiol Clin North Am 1974; 12:257-282
3. Taveras JM, Wood EH: Diagnostic Neuroradiology. (ed 2) Baltimore: Williams & Wilkins, vol 1, 1976

Gamut C-21

RADIOLUCENT LESION OR BONE DEFECT IN THE SKULL, SOLITARY OR MULTIPLE
(See Gamut C-20)

CONGENITAL OR DEVELOPMENTAL DEFECT
1. Congenital arachnoid cyst
*2. Congenital fibromatosis
*3. [Craniolacunia (lacunar skull)]
4. Dermoid
5. Ectopic intradiploic glial tissue
6. Encephalocele, meningoencephalocele, dermal sinus, median cleft face S., cranium bifidum
7. Epidermoid (primary cholesteatoma)

8. Fibrous dysplasia (incl. cortical)
9. Fontanelle
*10. Frontal fenestra
11. Hemangioma or arteriovenous malformation of bone or scalp
12. Inioindineal canal (emissary vein canal)
*13. Neurofibromatosis (eg, asterion or lambdoid suture defect, absent sphenoid wing)
*14. Pacchionian depression
*15. Parietal foramina
*16. Parietal thinning
*17. Venous lake or diploic channel
*18. Wide sutures (See C-40, C-41)

TRAUMATIC

*1. Burr hole; surgical defect; craniotomy
2. Fibrosing osteitis
*3. Fracture, simple or depressed
4. Hematoma (cephalhematoma, intradiploic, subdural); cephalhydrocele
5. Leptomeningeal cyst

INFLAMMATORY

1. Cholesteatoma
2. Hydatid disease
3. Mucocele of paranasal sinus
*4. Osteomyelitis, bacterial or fungal$_g$; abscess
*5. Sarcoidosis
*6. Syphilis, yaws
*7. Tuberculosis

NEOPLASTIC

1. Aneurysmal bone cyst
2. Chondroid lesion
3. Chordoma of clivus
4. Giant cell tumor (esp. complicating Paget's)
5. Glomus jugulare tumor
*6. Hemangioma, angiomatosis
7. Intracranial tumor with erosion

*8. Lymphoma$_g$, leukemia, chloroma
9. Malignant fibrous histiocytoma
10. Melanotic progonoma
11. Meningioma
*12. Metastasis (incl. neuroblastoma)
*13. Myeloma, plasmacytoma
14. Neoplasm of paranasal sinus or nasopharynx with erosion
15. Neurofibroma of bone or scalp
16. Sarcoma of bone (eg, Ewing's, osteosarcoma, chondrosarcoma, fibrosarcoma)
17. Skin or scalp tumor with invasion (eg, rodent ulcer)

MISCELLANEOUS
*1. Brown tumor of hyperparathyroidism
*2. Button sequestrum (See C-19)
3. Calvarial "doughnut", idiopathic
*4. Gaucher's disease; Niemann-Pick disease; Weber-Christian disease
5. Hemophilic pseudotumor
*6. Histiocytosis X$_g$
*7. Infantile cortical hyperostosis (Caffey's disease)
*8. Necrosis (eg, radiation therapy, electrical or thermal burn, postoperative bone flap necrosis)
9. Paget's disease (osteoporosis circumscripta)
*10. Parietal thinning, senile

*May be multiple.

References:
1. Du Boulay GH: Principles of X-ray Diagnosis of the Skull. (ed 2) London: Butterworths, 1980
2. Jacobson HG: Personal communication
3. Lane B: Erosions of the skull. Radiol Clin North Am 1974; 12:257-282
4. Lo Presti JM: Personal communication
5. Taveras JM, Wood EH: Diagnostic Neuroradiology. (ed 2) Baltimore: Williams & Wilkins, vol 1, 1976

ENLARGED, ERODED, OR DESTROYED SELLA TURCICA (INCLUDING INTRASELLAR OR PARASELLAR MASS ON CT OR MRI)

COMMON

1. Aneurysm or ectatic internal carotid artery (cavernous or suprasellar segment); carotid-cavernous fistula
2. Craniopharyngioma
3. Cretinism, hypothyroidism
4. Empty sella S.
5. Increased intracranial pressure, chronic (eg, obstructive hydrocephalus, dilated third ventricle, neoplasm, universal craniosynostosis)
6. Juxtasellar or suprasellar neoplasm, other (eg, meningioma, neurinoma of cranial nerves III to VI, optic chiasm glioma, epidermoid, dermoid, teratoma, hamartoma of tuber cinereum, hypothalamic glioma, germinoma, ectopic pinealoma)
7. [Osteoporosis; osteomalacia; hyperparathyroidism]
8. Pituitary adenoma (eg, chromophobe or eosinophilic adenoma, often with acromegaly or gigantism)

UNCOMMON

1. Abscess, pituitary
2. Arachnoid cyst, suprasellar or intrasellar, congenital or acquired (eg, after intracranial bleeding, infection, or with storage disease)
3. Basilar (transsphenoid) encephalocele
4. Benign neoplasm of skull base (eg, ossifying fibroma, osteochondroma, osteoma, chondroma)
5. Chordoma
6. Frontal lobe neoplasm
7. Histiocytosis X_g (often leading to diabetes insipidus)
8. Hypogonadism (incl. Turner S.)
9. Infundibular lesion (eg, metastasis, histiocytosis X_g, sarcoidosis)

10. Lymphoid hypophysitis (pituitary enlargement, usually with normal sella, in a postpartum woman with thyrotoxicosis)
11. Metastasis (esp. from lung or breast)
12. Mucocele of sphenoid sinus
13. Mucopolysaccharidoses (esp. Hurler S.); mucolipidosis
14. Neoplasm of sphenoid sinus or nasopharynx with local invasion (eg, carcinoma, angiofibroma, giant cell tumor)
15. Neurofibromatosis
16. Optic nerve neoplasm (eg, carcinoma, glioma, neurofibroma, meningioma)
17. Osteomyelitis, granuloma (eg, syphilis, tuberculosis, sarcoidosis, fungus disease$_g$)
18. Oxycephaly
19. Pituitary gland hypertrophy after adrenal ablation (Nelson S.) or with hypothyroidism
20. Pituitary neoplasm, other (eg, adenocarcinoma, carcinosarcoma, lymphomag, oncocytoma, prolactinoma, choristoma)
21. Postoperative change
22. Rathke cleft cyst

References:

1. Doyle FH: Radiology of the pituitary fossa. In: Lodge T, Steiner RE (eds): Recent Advances in Radiology. New York: Churchill Livingstone, 1979, vol 6, pp 121-143
2. DuBoulay GH: Principles of X-ray Diagnosis of the Skull. (ed 2) London: Butterworths, 1980
3. Kaufman B, Chamberlin WB Jr: The "empty" sella turcica. Acta Radiol 1970;13:413-425
4. Lee SH, Rao KC: Cranial Computed Tomography and MRI. (ed 2) New York: McGraw-Hill, 1987, pp 453-477
5. Newton TH, Potts DG: Radiology of the Skull and Brain. St. Louis: C.V. Mosby, 1971, vol 1, book 1, pp 372-402
6. Sage MR, Chan ESH, Reilly PL: The clinical and radiological features of the empty sella syndrome. Clin Radiol 1980; 31:513-519
7. Swischuk LE: Differential Diagnosis in Pediatric Radiology. Baltimore: Williams & Wilkins, 1984, pp 356-357
8. Taveras JM, Wood EH: Diagnostic Neuroradiology. (ed 2) Baltimore: Williams & Wilkins, 1976, vol 1, pp 65-89
9. Teasdale E, et al: The reliability of radiology in detecting prolactin-secreting pituitary microadenomas. Br J Radiol 1981; 54:556-571

C. Calvarium (Skull)

10. Tindall GT, Hoffman JC Jr: Evaluation of the abnormal sella turcica. Arch Intern Med 1980;140:1078-1083

Gamut C-23

SMALL SELLA TURCICA

COMMON
1. Decreased intracranial pressure (eg, brain atrophy, successful shunt for hydrocephalus)
2. Hypopituitarism; growth hormone deficiency
3. Normal variant

UNCOMMON
1. Cockayne S.
2. "Contracting skull" (postinflammatory or traumatic cerebral degeneration)
3. Cretinism, treated
4. Deprivation dwarfism
5. Fibrous dysplasia
6. Genetic (primordial) dwarfism
7. Microcephaly (See C-2)
8. Myotonic dystrophy
9. Prader-Willi S.
10. Radiation therapy during childhood
11. Sheehan S. (postpartum pituitary necrosis)
12. Trisomy 21 S. (Down S.)
13. Vestigial or dysplastic sella

References:
1. Newton TH, Potts DG: Radiology of the Skull and Brain. St. Louis: C.V. Mosby, 1971, vol 1, book 1, pp 371-372
2. Oh KS, Ledesma-Medina J, Bender TM: Practical Gamuts and Differential Diagnosis in Pediatric Radiology. Chicago: Year Book Medical Publ, 1982, p 8
3. Taybi H, Lachman RS: Radiology of Syndromes, Metabolic Disorders, and Skeletal Dysplasias. (ed 3) Chicago: Year Book Medical Publ, 1990, p 854

Gamut C-24

ABNORMAL SELLAR CONFIGURATION

J-Shaped Sella Turcica

COMMON
1. Hydrocephalus, mild arrested
2. Normal variant (5% of normal children)
3. Optic chiasm glioma

UNCOMMON
1. Achondroplasia
2. Cretinism
3. Hurler S. (gargoylism)
4. Neurofibromatosis (sphenoid dysplasia)
5. Pituitary tumor extending anteriorly
6. Subarachnoid cyst (intrasellar)
7. Suprasellar tumor

Elongated or Stretched Sella

1. Craniopharyngioma or other juxtasellar or suprasellar neoplasm (eg, meningioma)
2. Enlarging head (eg, storage diseases, chondro-dystrophies, hydrocephalus, megalencephaly)
3. Normal variant

Omega or Scooped Sella

1. Normal (unilateral)
2. Optic chiasm tumor (glioma, neurofibroma)
3. Pituitary fossa tumor

Dysplastic Sella

1. Neurofibromatosis

Reference:
1. Swischuk LE: Differential Diagnosis in Pediatric Radiology. Baltimore: Williams & Wilkins, 1984, pp 356-358

C. Calvarium (Skull)

Gamut C-25

FORAMEN MAGNUM ABNORMALITIES

Enlargement

COMMON
1. Arnold-Chiari malformation
2. Cervical-occipital meningocele or encephalocele
3. Dandy-Walker cyst; other posterior fossa cysts

UNCOMMON
1. Neoplasm of posterior fossa or upper cervical spine
2. Syringobulbia

Small or Irregular Foramen Magnum

1. Bilateral or unilateral occipitalization (fusion) of C1
   to base of skull
2. Chondrodystrophies
   a. Achondroplasia
   b. Achondrogenesis
   c. Diastrophic dysplasia
   d. Metatropic dysplasia
   e. Thanatophoric dysplasia

Reference:
1. Swischuk LE: Differential Diagnosis in Pediatric Radiology.
   Baltimore:Williams & Wilkins, 1984, pp 359-361

Gamut C-26

ENLARGEMENT OF THE JUGULAR CANAL

LESION WITHIN THE CANAL
1. Aneurysm of internal carotid artery
2. AV malformation
3. Glomus jugulare neoplasm
4. Neurinoma of cranial nerve IX, X, or XI
5. [Normal]

LESION ARISING OUTSIDE THE CANAL
1. Carcinoma of nasopharynx
2. Chondroma
3. Chordoma
4. Epidermoid
5. Meningioma
6. Metastasis
7. Osteoblastoma

References:
1. Crawford DB, Williams JP, Connaughton PN: Glomus jugulare tumors: The value of lateral tomography. American Roentgen Ray Society Scientific Exhibit, Atlanta, 1975
2. Newton TH, Hasso AN, Dillon WP: Modern Neuroradiology, vol 3. Computed Tomography of the Head and Neck. New York: Raven Press, 1988

Gamut C-27

EXPANSION OF THE MIDDLE FOSSA
(See Gamut C-28)

COMMON
1. Arachnoid cyst; temporal lobe agenesis or atrophy with overlying cerebrospinal fluid collection
2. Neoplasm of middle fossa, slow growing (eg, temporal lobe glioma, meningioma)
3. Subdural hematoma, chronic; hygroma

UNCOMMON
1. Neurofibromatosis
2. Oxycephaly with partial stenosis of sagittal and metopic sutures
3. Porencephalic cyst
4. Temporal horn hydrocephalus, localized

C. Calvarium (Skull)

EROSION OF THE MIDDLE FOSSA FLOOR
(See Gamuts C-27, B-28)

COMMON
1. Aneurysm of internal carotid artery (large); carotid-cavernous fistula
2. Arachnoid cyst
3. Chordoma
4. Glomus jugulare or vagale tumor
5. Malignant neoplasm of nasopharynx or paranasal sinus
6. Meningioma

UNCOMMON
1. Benign bone neoplasm (eg, chondroma, giant cell tumor)
2. [Congenital or postoperative defect]
3. Epidermoid, cholesteatoma
4. Histiocytosis X_g
5. Increased intracranial pressure, chronic
6. Metastasis
7. Neurinoma of fifth nerve (foramen ovale)
8. Neurofibromatosis
9. Temporal lobe glioma

References:
1. DuBoulay GH: Principles of X-ray Diagnosis of the Skull. (ed 2) London: Butterworths, 1980, pp 180-186
2. Hasso A, Vignaud J, La Masters DL: Pathology of the skull base and vault. In: Newton TH, Hasso AN, Dillon WP (eds): Modern Neuroradiology, vol 3. Computed Tomography of the Head and Neck. New York: Raven Press, 1988, pp 3.1-3.26
3. Newton TH, Potts DG: Radiology of the Skull and Brain. St. Louis: C.V. Mosby, 1971, vol 1, book 1, pp 311-313

Gamut C-29

EROSION OF THE SPHENOID WING
(See Gamut H-11)

COMMON
1. [Congenital defect, isolated or with neurofibromatosis]
*2. Meningioma

UNCOMMON
1. Benign bone neoplasm (eg, giant cell tumor, chondroma)
2. Chordoma
*3. Craniopharyngioma
4. Expansion of middle fossa (See C-27)
*5. Glioma (eg, optic)
6. Histiocytosis X_g
7. Increased intracranial pressure, chronic
8. Metastasis
9. Parasellar aneurysm
10. Pituitary tumor (esp. chromophobe adenoma)
11. Plexiform neurofibroma

* Lesser wing erosion; other lesions listed involve the greater wing.

References:
1. DuBoulay GH: Principles of X-ray Diagnosis of the Skull. (ed 2) London: Butterworths, 1980
2. Hasso A, Vignaud J, La Masters DL: Pathology of the skull base and vault. In: Newton TH, Hasso AN, Dillon WP (eds): Modern Neuroradiology, vol 3. Computed Tomography of the Head and Neck. New York: Raven Press, 1988, pp 3.1-3.26

Gamut C-30

EROSION OF THE PETROUS RIDGE, PYRAMID, OR APEX

COMMON
1. Acoustic neurinoma
2. Bone neoplasm, benign or malignant (eg, hemangioma, osteoblastoma, chondroma, chordoma)
3. Cholesteatoma, acquired or congenital (epidermoid)
4. Cholesterol granuloma
5. Metastasis

UNCOMMON
1. Aneurysm of intracavernous or intrapetrous carotid artery
2. Glioma
3. Glomus jugulare tumor
4. Histiocytosis X_g
5. Leptomeningeal cyst
6. Malignant neoplasm of nasopharynx (invasive)
7. Meningioma of Meckel's cave
8. Neurinoma of V, IX, or X nerve
9. Osteomyelitis, petrositis (Gradenigo S.)

References:
1. DuBoulay GH: Principles of X-ray Diagnosis of the Skull. (ed 2) London: Butterworths, 1980, pp 193-195
2. Livingstone PA: Differential diagnosis of radiolucent lesions of the temporal bone. Radiol Clin North Am 1974;12:571-583
3. Newton TH, Potts DG: Radiology of the Skull and Brain. St. Louis: C.V. Mosby, 1971, vol 1, book 1, pp 424, 447

Gamut C-31

EROSION OR WIDENING OF THE INTERNAL AUDITORY MEATUS

COMMON
1. Acoustic neurinoma
2. [Normal patulous canal]

UNCOMMON

1. Cholesteatoma, epidermoid
2. Cyst
3. Glioma of brain stem
4. Increased intracranial pressure, chronic hydrocephalus
5. Meningioma of cerebellopontine angle or petrous apex
6. Metastasis
7. Neurinoma of V or VII nerve
8. Neurofibromatosis
9. Vascular lesion (eg, aneurysm of internal auditory canal artery; AV malformation; hemangioma)

References:

1. Dubois PJ: Neuro-otology. In: Rosenberg RN (ed): The Clinical Neurosciences. New York: Churchill Livingstone, 1984, vol 4, p 672
2. DuBoulay GH: Principles of X-ray Diagnosis of the Skull (ed 2) London: Butterworths, 1980, pp 186-193
3. Newton TH, Potts DG: Radiology of the Skull and Brain. St. Louis: C.V. Mosby, 1971, vol 1, book 1, pp 442-446

Gamut C-32

DENSE TEMPORAL BONE LESION

COMMON

1. Fibrous dysplasia
2. Mastoiditis, chronic sclerotic

UNCOMMON

1. Craniometaphyseal dysplasia
2. Ossifying fibroma
3. Osteoblastic metastasis
4. Osteopetrosis
5. Osteosarcoma
6. Otodystrophies (See H-24)
7. Paget's disease (treated)

Reference:

1. Unger JM: Handbook of Head and Neck Imaging. New York: Churchill Livingstone, 1987, pp 160-161

C. Calvarium (Skull)

Gamut C-33

NEOPLASM INVOLVING THE TEMPORAL BONE

BENIGN

*1. Acoustic neurinoma (VIII nerve)
 2. Adenoma (soft tissue), ceruminous gland tumor of external auditory canal
*3. [Cholesterol granuloma]
*4. Epidermoid (congenital cholesteatoma)
 5. Exostosis of external auditory canal
 6. Giant cell tumor
 7. Glomus jugulare tumor; glomus tympanicum tumor
 8. Hemangioma
*9. [Histiocytosis X_g (esp. eosinophilic granuloma)]
10. Meningioma
11. Neurinoma of V, VII, IX, X, XI, or XII nerve
12. Osteoma, cancellous or compact

MALIGNANT

 1. Carcinoma of external auditory canal or rarely the middle ear
 2. Lymphoma$_g$, leukemia
*3. Metastasis (esp. from breast, lung, prostate, kidney, melanoma) or local extension from parotid carcinoma
 4. Myeloma
 5. Sarcoma (eg, rhabdomyosarcoma, fibrosarcoma, lymphosarcoma, osteosarcoma, chondrosarcoma, undifferentiated sarcoma)

* Common.

References:
 1. Unger JM: Handbook of Head and Neck Imaging. New York: Churchill Livingstone, 1987, pp 146-152
 2. Valvassori GE, Buckingham RA, Carter BL, Hanafee WN, Mafee MF: Head and Neck Imaging: New York: Thieme Medical Publ, 1988, pp 120-144

Gamut C-34

SKULL AND FACIAL BONES OF MEMBRANOUS ORIGIN

1. Facial bones, including mandible
2. Frontal bone
3. Occipital bone (upper squamosa)
4. Parietal bone
5. Pterygoid (medial plate)
6. Temporal bone (squamosal and tympanic parts)
7. Vomer

Reference:
1. Greenfield GB: Radiology of Bone Diseases. (ed 5) Philadelphia: Lippincott, 1990

Gamut C-35

NORMAL SKULL VARIANT

COMMON
1. Arterial groove (eg, middle meningeal)
2. [Artifact (eg, hair braid, rubber band, skin fold, EEG paste, surgical tape or dressing, skin laceration with air trapping)]
3. Convolutional impressions
4. Dural sinus (eg, transverse or sigmoid sinus)
5. Emissary vein, venous lake, diploic channel, sinus groove
6. Fontanelle
7. Metopic suture, mendosal suture
8. Pacchionian granulation
9. Sutural (wormian) bones; interparietal sutures; atypical suture line
10. Torcular Herophili

UNCOMMON

1. Cruciate ridge
2. Inioindineal canal
3. Interparietal bone
4. Occipital fissure; posterior parietal fissure
5. Parietal foramina
6. Parietal thinning
7. Unfused planum sphenoidale

References:

1. Swischuk LE: The normal pediatric skull: Variations and artifacts. Radiol Clin North Am 1972;10:227-290
2. Tomsick TA: Gamut: Normal skull variant that may simulate a fracture. Semin Roentgenol 1978;13:3

Subgamut C-35A

NORMAL SKULL VARIANTS THAT MAY SIMULATE A FRACTURE

1. Arterial groove (eg, meningeal vessels, middle temporal branch of superficial temporal artery, deep temporal branches of internal maxillary artery, supraorbital artery)
2. Artifact or soft tissue alteration (eg, skin laceration, skin fold, air trapped beneath skin, matted hair, hair braid, rubber band, tape, dressing, linen)
3. Emissary vein, venous lake, diploic channel, sinus groove
4. Fissure, synchondrosis, suture
   a. Cerebellar synchondrosis
   b. Coronal suture
   c. Innominate synchondrosis
   d. Interparietal suture
   e. Intersphenoid synchondrosis
   f. Lambdoid suture
   g. Lateral fissures of the foramen magnum

    h. Lateral interparietal fissure
    i. Lateral sphenoidal suture
    j. Median occipital fissure
    k. Mendosal suture
    l. Metopic suture
    m. Occipitomastoid suture
    n. Parietal fissure
    o. Parietomastoid suture
    p. Spheno-occipital synchondrosis
    q. Squamosal suture
    r. Transverse occipital suture
    s. Unfused planum sphenoidale
5. Wormian (sutural) bone

References:

1. Allen WE, Kier EL, Rothman SLG: Pitfalls in the evaluation of skull trauma. Radiol Clin North Am 1973;11:479-503
2. Keats TE: Atlas of Normal Roentgen Variants That May Simulate Disease. (ed 4) Chicago: Year Book Medical Publ, 1988
3. Swischuk LE: The normal pediatric skull: Variations and artifacts. Radiol Clin North Am 1972;10:277-290
4. Tomsick TA: Gamut: Normal skull variant that may simulate a fracture. Semin Roentgenol 1978;13:3

Gamut C-36

MULTIPLE WORMIAN (SUTURAL) BONES

COMMON
1. Cleidocranial dysplasia
2. Cretinism, hypothyroidism
3. Hypophosphatasia
4. Normal; idiopathic
5. Osteogenesis imperfecta
6. Progeria
7. Pyknodysostosis

UNCOMMON

1. Aminopterin fetopathy
2. Cerebrohepatorenal S. (Zellweger S.)
3. Chondrodysplasia punctata (Conradi's disease)
4. Familial idiopathic osteoarthropathy (Currarino S.)
5. Hajdu-Cheney S. (idiopathic acro-osteolysis)
6. Hallermann-Streiff S.
7. Hydrocephalus, infantile
8. Kinky-hair S. (Menkes S.); copper deficiency
9. Metaphyseal chondrodysplasia (Jansen)
10. Osteopetrosis, infantile type; sclerosteosis
11. Pachydermoperiostosis
12. Prader-Willi S.
13. [Rickets]
14. Trisomy 21 S. (Down S.)

References:

1. Cremin B, Goodman H, Spranger J, et al: Wormian bones in osteogenesis imperfecta and other disorders. Skeletal Radiol 1982;8:35-38
2. Greenfield GB: Radiology of Bone Diseases. (ed 5) Philadelphia: Lippincott, 1990
3. Kozlowski K, Beighton P: Gamut Index of Skeletal Dysplasias. Berlin: Springer-Verlag, 1984, pp 35-36
4. Pryles CV, Khan AJ: Wormian bones. Am J Dis Child 1979; 133:380-382
5. Taybi H, Lachman RS: Radiology of Syndromes, Metabolic Disorders, and Skeletal Dysplasias. (ed 3) Chicago: Year Book Medical Publ, 1990, p 855

Gamut C-37

DELAYED OR DEFECTIVE CRANIAL OSSIFICATION

TRANSIENT
(Spontaneous correction before 3 years of age)

1. Aminopterin fetopathy
2. Cerebrohepatorenal S. (Zellweger S.)

3. Congenital lacunar skull
4. Congenital scalp defect S.
5. Cutis laxa; Ehlers-Danlos S.
6. Hypophosphatasia
7. Kinky-hair S. (Menkes S.)
8. Metaphyseal chondrodysplasia (Jansen)
9. Mucopolysaccharidoses (eg, Hunter, Hurler)
10. Osteogenesis imperfecta
11. Rubinstein-Taybi S.
12. Silver-Russell S.
13. Trisomy 13 S.
14. Trisomy 18 S.
15. Trisomy 21 S. (Down S.)

INTERMEDIATE
(Spontaneous correction between 3 and 10 years)
1. Cretinism, hypothyroidism
2. Otopalatodigital S.
3. Pachydermoperiostosis
4. Progeria
5. Rickets

PROTRACTED
(Persistence beyond 10 years of age)
1. Cleidocranial dysplasia
2. Cranium bifidum occultum
3. Dermal sinus
4. Encephalocele
5. Frontonasal dysplasia
6. Hypertelorism with Sprengel's deformity
7. Oculo-mandibulo-facial S. (Hallermann-Streiff S.)
8. Parietal foramina; occipital foramina
9. Parietal thinning
10. Pyknodysostosis
11. Stanescu dysostosis
12. Tubular stenosis (Kenny-Caffey S.)

Reference:
1. Dorst JP: Personal communication

C. Calvarium (Skull)

Gamut C-38

SMALL ANTERIOR FONTANELLE

1. Craniosynostosis, primary
2. Craniosynostosis, secondary (eg, chronic anemia$_g$, rickets, hypophosphatasia)
3. Decreased intracranial pressure (eg, brain atrophy, shunted hydrocephalus)
4. Normal variant

Reference:
1. Swischuk LE: Differential Diagnosis in Pediatric Radiology. Baltimore: Williams & Wilkins, 1984, p 362

Gamut C-39

CONGENITAL SYNDROMES WITH LARGE ANTERIOR FONTANELLE OR DELAYED CLOSURE OF FONTANELLES

COMMON
1. Cleidocranial dysplasia
2. Cretinism, hypothyroidism
3. Hypophosphatasia
4. Intrauterine growth failure or infection (eg, rubella S.)
5. Normal (esp. in premature)
6. Osteogenesis imperfecta
7. Rickets, severe

UNCOMMON
1. Aase S.
2. Aminopterin fetopathy
3. Cerebrohepatorenal S. (Zellweger S.)
4. Chondrodysplasia punctata (Conradi's disease)
5. Congenital scalp defect S. (aplasia cutis)

6. Cranium bifidum with lacunar skull
7. Cutis laxa
8. Familial idiopathic osteoarthropathy
9. Fetal hydantoin S.
10. Fetal primidone S.
11. G syndrome
12. Goldenhar S.
13. Greig cephalopolysyndactyly S.
14. Hallermann-Streiff S.
15. Hypochondroplasia
16. Lenz-Majewski hyperostotic dwarfism
17. Osteodysplasty (Melnick-Needles S.)
18. Otopalatodigital S.
19. Progeria
20. Pyknodysostosis
21. Rubinstein-Taybi S.
22. Silver-Russell S.
23. Trisomy 13 S.
24. Trisomy 21 S. (Down S.)
25. Tubular stenosis (Kenny-Caffey S.)
26. Winchester S.

References:

1. Dorst J: Radiological Society of North America Scientific Exhibit, 1972
2. Felson B (ed): Dwarfs and other little people. Semin Roentgenol 1973;8:133-263
3. Jones KL: Smith's Recognizable Patterns of Human Malformation. Philadelphia: W.B. Saunders, 1988
4. Swischuk LE: Differential Diagnosis in Pediatric Radiology. Baltimore: Williams & Wilkins, 1984, p 362
5. Taybi H, Lachman RS: Radiology of Syndromes, Metabolic Disorders, and Skeletal Dysplasias. (ed 3) Chicago: Year Book Medical Publ, 1990, p 853

Gamut C-40

DELAYED CLOSURE AND/OR INCOMPLETE OSSIFICATION OF SUTURES

COMMON

1. Cleidocranial dysplasia
2. Cretinism, hypothyroidism
3. Hydrocephalus
4. Increased intracranial pressure (esp. brain neoplasm)
5. Infiltration of sutures (eg, metastatic neuroblastoma, leukemia)
6. Intrauterine growth failure or infection (eg, rubella S.)
7. Normal, prematurity
8. Osteogenesis imperfecta
9. Osteoporosis, severe
10. Rickets
11. Trisomy 21 S. (Down S.)

UNCOMMON

1. Aminopterin fetopathy
2. Cerebrohepatorenal S. (Zellweger S.)
3. Cranium bifidum
4. Diencephalic S.
5. Familial idiopathic osteoarthropathy (Currarino S.)
6. Fetal primidone S.
7. Hajdu-Cheney S. (idiopathic acro-osteolysis)
8. Hallermann-Streiff S.
9. Hyperparathyroidism, primary infantile or secondary (renal osteodystrophy)
10. Hypoparathyroidism
11. Hypophosphatasia
12. Neurofibromatosis (bone defect along lambdoid suture)
13. Pachydermoperiostosis
14. Progeria
15. Prolonged parenteral hyperalimentation
16. Psychosocial (deprivation) dwarfism

C. Calvarium (Skull)

17. Pyknodysostosis
18. Rubinstein-Taybi S.
19. Silver-Russell S.
20. Vitamin A deficiency or intoxication
21. Winchester S.

References:
1. Newton TH, Potts DG: Radiology of the Skull and Brain. St. Louis: C.V. Mosby, 1971, vol 1, book 1, pp 232-236
2. Taybi H, Lachman RS: Radiology of Syndromes, Metabolic Disorders, and Skeletal Dysplasias. (ed 3) Chicago: Year Book Medical Publ, 1990, pp 854-855

Gamut C-41

SEPARATION OR INFILTRATION OF SKULL SUTURES IN AN INFANT OR CHILD
(See Gamut C-40)

COMMON
1. Brain abscess, cerebritis
2. Brain neoplasm (eg, pinealoma, medulloblastoma)
3. Cerebral edema, hemorrhage, or contusion
4. Hydrocephalus (See B-48, B-48A)
5. Incomplete ossification adjacent to sutures (See C-40)
6. Increased intracranial pressure, other causes (See B-47)
7. Lead poisoning, other encephalopathy
8. Leukemia, lymphoma$_g$
9. Meningitis, meningoencephalitis
10. Neuroblastoma, metastatic
11. Normal (esp. prematurity)
12. Subdural hematoma or hygroma

UNCOMMON
1. Hydranencephaly
2. Hypervitaminosis A
3. Intracranial cyst
4. Megalencephaly
5. Pseudotumor cerebri
6. Rebound growth of brain and body after treatment for hypothyroidism or deprivation dwarfism

References:
1. Swischuk LE: Differential Diagnosis in Pediatric Radiology. Baltimore: Williams & Wilkins, 1984, pp 347-348
2. Swischuk LE: The growing skull. Semin Roentgenol 1974; 9:115-124

Gamut C-42

DECREASED OR ABSENT CONVOLUTIONAL MARKINGS

COMMON
1. Cerebral atrophy
2. Normal to age 3 years
3. Shunted hydrocephalus

UNCOMMON
1. Cretinism, hypothyroidism
2. Deprivation dwarfism
3. Failure to thrive, severe

Reference:
1. Swischuk LE: Differential Diagnosis in Pediatric Radiology. Baltimore: Williams & Wilkins, 1984, pp 352-354

Gamut C-43

INCREASED CONVOLUTIONAL MARKINGS

COMMON
1. Craniosynostosis, primary (localized or universal)
2. Increased intracranial pressure, chronic (eg, neoplasm, cyst, hydrocephalus) (See B-47, B-48)
3. Lacunar skull (craniolacunia, lückenschädel)
4. Normal

UNCOMMON
1. Cloverleaf skull
2. Craniometaphyseal dysplasia
3. Craniosynostosis, secondary (eg, healing rickets, hypophosphatasia, hypercalcemia, hyperthyroidism, chronic anemia$_g$)

Reference:
1. Swischuk LE: Differential Diagnosis in Pediatric Radiology. Baltimore: Williams & Wilkins, 1984, pp 352-354

Gamut C-44

INCREASED SIZE OF THE VASCULAR GROOVES OF THE SKULL

COMMON
1. AV malformation
2. Hemangioma of skull
3. Meningioma

UNCOMMON
1. Collateral circulation (eg, thrombosis of a venous sinus, occlusion of internal carotid artery)
2. Fibrous dysplasia
3. Metastasis (eg, thyroid carcinoma, hypernephroma)
4. Pacchionian granulations
5. Paget's disease
6. Sarcoma or other malignant neoplasm of skull

Gamut C-45

"HAIR ON END" OR "SUNBURST" PATTERN IN THE SKULL

Generalized ("Hair on End")

COMMON
1. Congenital hemolytic anemias$_g$ (eg, thalassemia, sickle cell disease, hereditary spherocytosis, elliptocytosis)

UNCOMMON
1. Congenital cyanotic heart disease with secondary polycythemia
2. Hypernephroma with increased erythropoiesis
3. Iron deficiency anemia, severe
4. Leukemia, lymphoma$_g$
5. Multiple myeloma
6. Polycythemia vera
7. Red cell enzyme deficiencies with secondary reticulocytosis (eg, pyruvate kinase, hexokinase, glucose-6-phosphate dehydrogenase)

Localized ("Sunburst" Spiculations)

COMMON
1. Hemangioma
2. Meningioma
3. Metastasis (esp. neuroblastoma, prostate, breast)

UNCOMMON
1. Ewing's sarcoma
2. Osteosarcoma

References:
1. Greenfield GB: Radiology of Bone Diseases. (ed 5) Philadelphia: Lippincott, 1990
2. Kohler A, Zimmer EA: Borderlands of the Normal and Early Pathologic in Skeletal Radiology. New York: Grune & Stratton, 1968, p 202
3. Silverman FN: Caffey's Pediatric X-ray Diagnosis (ed 8) Chicago: Year Book Medical Publ, 1985, pp 79-85
4. Swischuk LE: Differential Diagnosis in Pediatric Radiology. Baltimore: Williams & Wilkins, 1984, pp 341-343
5. Wilson JD, et al: Harrison's Principles of Internal Medicine. (ed 12) New York: McGraw-Hill, 1991

C. Calvarium (Skull)

H

Head and Neck
(See Section "M"
for MRI of the Head
and Neck)

H

H

Gamut H-1

MALFORMATION OF THE ORBIT

COMMON
1. Craniosynostosis (See C-1)
2. Enucleation in childhood, traumatic or surgical
3. Fibrous dysplasia, leontiasis ossea

UNCOMMON
1. Anophthalmos, microphthalmos
2. Cerebral atrophy and mental retardation (round orbits)
3. Encroachment from adjacent mass (eg, frontal sinus mucocele, antral neoplasm or cyst)
4. Forebrain hypoplasia, arhinencephaly S. (round orbits)
5. Hypertelorism (eg, Apert S., Crouzon S., Treacher Collins S.) (See H-3, H-3A)
6. Hypotelorism (See H-2)
7. Neoplasm (eg, neurofibroma)
8. Neurofibromatosis
9. Radiation therapy

Gamut H-2

HYPOTELORISM (DECREASED INTERORBITAL DISTANCE)

1. Craniotelencephalic dysplasia
2. Cyclops
3. Holoprosencephaly (arhinencephaly)
4. Myotonic dystrophy
5. Oculo-dento-osseous dysplasia
6. Postaxial acrofacial dysostosis (Miller S.)
7. Sagittal craniosynostosis
8. Trigonocephaly (premature closure of metopic suture)

9. Trisomy 13 S.
10. Trisomy 21 S. (Down S.)
11. Williams S. (idiopathic hypercalcemia)

References:

1. Swischuk LE: Differential Diagnosis in Pediatric Radiology. Baltimore: Williams & Wilkins, 1984, p 387
2. Taybi H, Lachman RS: Radiology of Syndromes, Metabolic Disorders, and Skeletal Dysplasias. (ed 3) Chicago: Year Book Medical Publ, 1990, p 844

Gamut H-3

HYPERTELORISM

1. Anterior meningocele or encephalocele; cranium bifidum
2. Congenital syndromes (See H-3A)
3. Craniosynostosis of coronal sutures
4. Dermoid (midline)
5. Fibrous dysplasia, leontiasis ossea
6. Hydrocephalus in growth period, severe (overgrowth of lesser wing of sphenoid)
7. Idiopathic
8. Mucocele
9. Nasal tumor

Subgamut H-3A

CONGENITAL SYNDROMES WITH HYPERTELORISM

COMMON
1. Cleidocranial dysplasia
2. Craniofacial dysostosis (Crouzon S.)

3. Familial hypertelorism; normal variant
4. Greig cephalopolysyndactyly S.
5. Median cleft face S. (median cleft nose and palate)
6. Treacher Collins S. (mandibulofacial dysostosis)

UNCOMMON

1. Aarskog S.
2. Acrocephalosyndactyly (Apert, Pfeiffer, Saethre-Chotzen types)
3. Acrodysostosis
4. Aminopterin fetopathy
5. Basal cell nevus S. (Gorlin S.)
6. Beckwith-Wiedemann S.
7. Bird-headed dwarfism (Seckel S.)
8. Blackfan-Diamond S.
9. Cat-eye S.
10. Cat's cry S. (cri du chat S.)
11. Cerebral gigantism (Sotos S.)
12. Chondrodysplasia punctata (Conradi's disease)
13. Chromosome syndromes (4p-, 4p+, 18p-)
14. Cloverleaf skull
15. Coffin-Lowry S.
16. Cornelia de Lange S.
17. Craniometaphyseal dysplasia
18. Cryptophthalmia S. (Fraser S.)
19. Di George S.
20. Dubowitz S.
21. Dyssegmental dysplasia
22. Fetal hydantoin S.
23. G syndrome
24. Hypertelorism-hypospadias S.
25. Larsen S.
26. Lenz-Majewski hyperostotic dwarfism
27. LEOPARD S. (lentiginosis S.)
28. Metaphyseal chondrodysplasia (Jansen)
29. Noonan S.
30. Oro-facio-digital S.
31. Osteoglophonic dwarfism
32. Osteopetrosis

33. Otopalatodigital S.
34. Pena-Shokeir S.
35. Potter S.
36. Pterygium syndromes
37. Roberts S.
38. Robinow S.
39. Rubinstein-Taybi S.
40. Sclerosteosis
41. Sjögren-Larsson S.
42. Spondyloepiphyseal dysplasia congenita
43. [Thalassemia]
44. Waardenburg S.
45. Warfarin embryopathy
46. Whistling face S. (Freeman-Sheldon S.)
47. XXXXX S.
48. XXXXY S.

References:

1. Jones KL: Smith's Recognizable Patterns of Human Malformation. (ed 3) Philadelphia: W.B. Saunders, 1988
2. MacPherson RI, Wan R, Reed MH: Hypertelorism. American Roentgen Ray Society Scientific Exhibit, San Francisco, 1974
3. Swischuk LE: Differential Diagnosis in Pediatric Radiology. Baltimore: Williams & Wilkins, 1984, p 388
4. Taybi H, Lachman RS: Radiology of Syndromes, Metabolic Disorders, and Skeletal Dysplasias. (ed 3) Chicago: Year Book Medical Publ, 1990, p 844

Gamut H-4

SMALL ORBIT AND/OR OPTIC CANAL

COMMON

1. Enucleation in childhood
2. Optic nerve atrophy
3. Radiation therapy

UNCOMMON

1. Anophthalmos, microphthalmos (eg, Hallermann-Streiff S., oculovertebral S.- unilateral, trisomy 13 S., oculo-dento-osseous dysplasia)
2. Congenital underdevelopment of globe and face (unilateral)
3. Craniosynostosis of coronal suture
4. Encroachment from adjacent mass (eg, frontal sinus mucocele or neoplasm; antral neoplasm or cyst)
5. Forebrain hypoplasia syndromes with hypotelorism (See H-2)
6. Neurofibromatosis (orbital dysplasia)
7. Osteitis (eg, from sphenoid sinusitis)
8. Osteoblastic bone lesion or hyperostosis with encroachment on orbit (eg, meningioma, fibrous dysplasia, Paget's disease, osteopetrosis, craniometaphyseal dysplasia, hypercalcemia, thalassemia)

References:

1. Newton TH, Potts DG: Radiology of the Skull and Brain. St. Louis: C.V. Mosby, vol 1, book 2, 1971, pp 469-470, 502-506
2. Swischuk LE: Differential Diagnosis in Pediatric Radiology. Baltimore: Williams & Wilkins, 1984, pp 384-387
3. Taybi H, Lachman RS: Radiology of Syndromes, Metabolic Disorders, and Skeletal Dysplasias. (ed 3) Chicago: Year Book Medical Publ, 1990, pp 845-846

Gamut H-5

LARGE ORBIT

COMMON

1. Coronal craniosynostosis with elevation of orbit
2. Exophthalmos (eg, thyrotoxicosis)
3. Pseudotumor of orbit
4. Tumor, intraconal (eg, hemangioma, optic nerve glioma, neurofibroma, retinoblastoma, metastasis) or extraconal

UNCOMMON

1. Congenital glaucoma (buphthalmos, hydrophthalmos)
2. Congenital serous cyst (often associated with anophthalmos or microphthalmos)
3. Histiocytosis X_g
4. Hypoplastic maxilla
5. Lymphoma$_g$, Burkitt's tumor
6. Neurofibromatosis (orbital dysplasia)
7. [Small contralateral orbit]
8. Varix of orbital vein

References:

1. Newton TH, Potts DG: Radiology of the Skull and Brain. St. Louis: C.V. Mosby, vol 1, book 2, 1971, pp 470-473
2. Taybi H, Lachman RS: Radiology of Syndromes, Metabolic Disorders, and Skeletal Dysplasias. (ed 3) Chicago: Year Book Medical Publ, 1990, p 845

Gamut H-6

LESIONS INVOLVING THE ORBIT
(See Gamuts H-7 to H-9, H-12)

ARISING WITHIN THE ORBIT

Intraocular or Intraconal Mass

1. Choroidal osteoma
2. Hamartoma (tuberous sclerosis)
*3. Infiltration of retrobulbar fat and intraorbital soft tissues (eg, amyloidosis, Erdheim-Chester disease)
*4. Intraocular foreign body
*5. Melanoma
*6. Meningioma of optic nerve
7. Metastasis (esp. lung, breast)
8. Neurinoma of optic nerve; neurofibroma of cranial nerve III, IV, or V
9. Ophthalmic artery aneurysm

*10. Optic glioma
 11. Optic neuritis
*12. Pseudotumor
 13. Retinoblastoma
 14. Sarcoma
 15. Vascular lesion (eg, cavernous or capillary heman-
     gioma, hemangiopericytoma, lymphangioma, venous
     angioma, orbital varices)

Extraconal or Muscle Mass
 1. Dacryocystitis
 2. Dermoid cyst; epidermoid
*3. Graves' disease
 4. Hematoma
*5. Lacrimal gland tumor
*6. Lymphoma$_g$, Burkitt's tumor
*7. Meningioma
*8. Metastasis
 9. Orbital myositis
*10. Pseudotumor
 11. Rhabdomyosarcoma
*12. Trauma
*13. Vascular lesion (eg, hemangioma, AV fistula, lymph-
     angioma, hemangioblastoma, hemangiopericytoma,
     varices)

**ARISING EXTRAORBITALLY OR
EXTRACRANIALLY
(EG, NASOPHARYNX, NASAL CAVITY,
PARANASAL SINUS, ORBITAL BONE, OR
INFRATEMPORAL FOSSA)**
 1. Bone neoplasm, benign (eg, osteoma*, osteochon-
    droma, chondroma, aneurysmal bone cyst, ossifying
    fibroma)
*2. Bone neoplasm, malignant (eg, sarcoma, myeloma,
    metastasis)
*3. Carcinoma of paranasal sinus, nasal cavity, or skin
 4. Craniofacial malformations
 5. Esthesioneuroblastoma of nasal cavity

6. Fibrous dysplasia (leontiasis ossea); other bone dysplasia
7. Granulomatous disease (eg, tuberculosis, sarcoidosis, Wegener's granulomatosis, lethal midline granuloma)
8. Histiocytosis X_g
9. Hydatid disease
10. Juvenile angiofibroma (esp. in pterygopalatine fossa)
*11. Lymphoma$_g$, Burkitt's tumor
12. Mucocele
13. Neurofibromatosis
*14. Orbital abscess or cellulitis (eg, from sinusitis or eyelid infection)
*15. Osteomyelitis
16. Osteopetrosis
*17. Paget's disease
18. Sinus neoplasm (eg, carcinoma, inverting papilloma)
*19. Trauma (incl. foreign body)

ARISING INTRACRANIALLY WITH SECONDARY INVOLVEMENT OF ORBIT

1. Aneurysm of internal carotid artery
2. Carotid-cavernous fistula
3. Chiasmatic arachnoiditis
4. Chordoma
5. Craniopharyngioma
6. Encephalomeningocele
7. Hypothalamic tumor
*8. Meningioma (anterior or middle fossa)
9. Optic glioma
10. Pituitary adenoma

*Common.

References:

1. Arger PH, Mishkin MM, Nenninger RH: An approach to orbital lesions. AJR 1972;115:595-606
2. Bryan RN, Craig JA: The eye: CT of the orbit. In: Bergeron RT, Osborn AG, Som PM: Head and Neck Imaging Excluding the Brain. St. Louis: C.V. Mosby, 1984, pp 575-616
3. Eisenberg RL: Clinical Imaging: An Atlas of Differential Diagnosis. (ed 2) Rockville, MD: Aspen Publishers, 1992, pp 966-973

4. Forbes GS, Sheedy PF II, Waller RR: Orbital tumors evaluated by computed tomography. Radiology 1980;136:101

5. Hesselink JR, Davis KR, Weber AL, et al: Radiological evaluation of orbital metastases, with emphasis on computed tomography. Radiology 1980;137:363

6. Hilal SK, Trokel SL: Computerized tomography of the orbit using thin sections. Semin Roentgenol 1977;12:137-147

7. Levine HL, Ferris EJ, Lessel S, et al: The neuroradiologic evaluation of "optic neuritis." AJR 1975;125:702-716

8. MacPherson P: The radiology of orbital meningioma. Clin Radiol 1979; 30:105

Gamut H-7

CT CHARACTERISTICS OF ORBITAL MASSES IN CHILDREN

	Location					Bone destruction	Calcification	Extension		Attenuation		Enhancement
	Preseptal	Extraconal	Intraconal	Muscle only	Orbital expansion			Intracranial	Facial	High	Low	
Optic nerve glioma	+/-		+		+			+				+
Rhabdomyosarcoma	+/-	+				+	-	+	+			+
2° Neuroblastoma	+	+				+	+	+	+	+		+
Lymphangioma	+	+	+		+						mixed	+/-
Hemangioma	+	+	+		+						mixed	+ irregular
Histiocytosis X	+/-	+				+	+	+	+			+
Infection	+	+							+			+
Leukemia	+	+		+		+						
Lymphoma	+	+				+			+	+		+
Dermoid	+	+	+		+					mixed		
Pseudotumor	+	+	+	+								

Reference:

1. Lallemand DP, Brasch RC, Char DH, Norman D: Orbital tumors in children. Characterisation by computed tomography. Radiology 1984;151:85-88 (slightly modified)

Gamut H-8

BONY DEFECT, EROSION, OR
RADIOLUCENT LESION OF THE ORBIT
(See Gamuts H-6, H-12)

COMMON
1. Extrinsic tumor invading orbit (eg, meningioma; carcinoma or lymphoma of nasopharynx, nasal cavity, or paranasal sinus; carcinoma of skin or eyelid)
2. Metastasis (eg, breast, lung, neuroblastoma, Ewing's sarcoma)
3. Mucocele
4. Osteomyelitis usually secondary to sinusitis
5. Primary orbital neoplasm (eg, hemangioma, hemangioblastoma, lacrimal gland carcinoma, dermoid, epidermoid, optic glioma, neurofibroma, melanoma, retinoblastoma, rhabdomyosarcoma, lymphoma$_g$, Burkitt's tumor)

UNCOMMON
1. Encephalomeningocele
2. Histiocytosis X$_g$
3. Juvenile angiofibroma
4. Multiple myeloma
5. Neurofibromatosis (orbital dysplasia) - "empty orbit"
6. Primary bone tumor

References:
1. Jacobs L, Weisberg LA, Kinkel WR: Computerized Tomography of the Orbit and Sella Turcica. New York: Raven Press, 1980
2. Newton TH, Potts DG: Radiology of the Skull and Brain. St. Louis: C.V. Mosby, vol 1, book 2, 1971, pp 476-482

SCLEROSIS AND THICKENING OF THE ORBITAL ROOF OR WALLS

COMMON

1. Fibrous dysplasia, leontiasis ossea
2. Meningioma
3. Osteitis secondary to chronic sinusitis or mucocele
4. Paget's disease

UNCOMMON

1. Craniometaphyseal dysplasia; frontometaphyseal dysplasia
2. Dermoid
3. Histiocytosis X_g
4. Infantile cortical hyperostosis (Caffey's disease)
5. Lacrimal gland carcinoma
6. Lymphoma$_g$
7. Osteoblastic metastasis (eg, breast, prostate)
8. Osteoma
9. Osteopetrosis
10. Osteosarcoma
11. Radiation therapy
12. Thalassemia

Reference:

1. Newton TH, Potts DG: Radiology of the Skull and Brain. St. Louis: C.V. Mosby, vol 1, book 2, 1971, pp 482-485

Gamut H-10

NARROWED SUPERIOR ORBITAL (SPHENOIDAL) FISSURE

COMMON

1. Fibrous dysplasia
2. Normal variant; congenital asymmetry or narrowing
3. Paget's disease

UNCOMMON
1. Bone neoplasm (eg, osteoma, osteoblastic metastasis)
2. Meningioma with hyperostosis
3. Osteitis secondary to chronic sinusitis
4. Osteopetrosis
5. Thalassemia

References:
1. Newton TH, Potts DG: Radiology of the Skull and Brain. St. Louis: C.V. Mosby, vol 1, book 2, 1971, pp 521-524
2. Shapiro R, Robinson F: Alterations of the sphenoidal fissure produced by local and systemic processes. AJR 1967;101: 814-827

Gamut H-11

ENLARGED SUPERIOR ORBITAL (SPHENOIDAL) FISSURE (EROSION AND WIDENING)

COMMON
1. Aneurysm of intracavernous portion of internal carotid artery
2. Normal asymmetry
3. Pituitary tumor (esp. chromophobe adenoma)

UNCOMMON
1. Carotid-cavernous fistula
2. Chordoma (parasellar)
3. Craniopharyngioma
4. Extension from orbital or infraorbital mass (eg, hemangioma, AV malformation, optic glioma, juvenile xanthogranuloma, lymphoma$_g$, Burkitt's tumor, neuroblastoma) or from paranasal sinus malignancy
5. Histiocytosis X$_g$
6. Increased intracranial pressure, long-standing
7. Meningioma, orbital or intracranial

8. Metastatic carcinoma to sphenoid wing
9. Middle fossa mass (eg, infratemporal chronic sub-dural hematoma or hygroma; arachnoid cyst with temporal lobe agenesis; temporal lobe astrocytoma)
10. Mucocele of sphenoid sinus
11. Neurofibroma
12. Neurofibromatosis (orbital dysplasia)
13. Orbital varix
14. Posterior orbital encephalocele
15. Pseudotumor of orbit
16. Superior orbital fissure S. (impairment of cranial nerves III, IV, and VI associated with sphenoid sinusitis)

References:
1. DuBoulay GH: Principles of X-ray Diagnosis of the Skull. (ed 2) London: Butterworths, 1980
2. Newton TH, Potts DG: Radiology of the Skull and Brain. St. Louis: C.V. Mosby, vol 1, book 2, 1971, pp 508-521

Gamut H-12

LOCALIZED BONY DEFECT OR EROSION ABOUT THE OPTIC CANAL
(See Gamuts H-8, H-13)

COMMON
1. Aneurysm of internal carotid artery (cavernous portion)
2. Malignant neoplasm arising in orbit, sphenoid sinus, or nasal cavity
3. Pituitary adenoma

UNCOMMON
1. Craniopharyngioma
2. Granuloma (eg, tuberculosis, sarcoidosis)
3. Histiocytosis X_g
4. Metastasis

5. Mucocele of sphenoid sinus
6. Neoplasm of anterior fossa (eg, meningioma, astrocytoma, glioma)
7. Neurofibroma, neurofibromatosis
8. Surgical defect

Reference:
1. Newton TH, Potts DG: Radiology of the Skull and Brain. St. Louis: C.V. Mosby, vol 1, book 2, 1971, pp 496-501

Gamut H-13

OPTIC CANAL ENLARGEMENT (OVER 6.5 MM IN DIAMETER) (See Gamuts H-12, H-14)

COMMON
1. Glioma of optic nerve
2. Meningioma of optic nerve sheath
3. Metastasis
4. Neurofibromatosis with or without optic neurofibroma or glioma

UNCOMMON
1. Aneurysm of ophthalmic artery or cavernous portion of internal carotid artery
2. AV malformation with ophthalmic artery involvement
3. Carcinoma of ethmoid or sphenoid sinus
4. Granuloma (eg, tuberculosis, sarcoidosis)
5. Increased intracranial pressure
6. Mucocele of sphenoid sinus
7. Mucopolysaccharidoses (esp. Hurler S.)
8. Pituitary adenoma or craniopharyngioma extending anteriorly
9. Pseudotumor of orbit
10. Retinoblastoma with intracranial extension

References:
1. Burgener FA, Kormano M: Differential Diagnosis in Conventional Radiology. (ed 2) New York: Thieme Medical Publ, 1991, pp 156-158
2. Lloyd GAS: Radiology of the Orbit. Philadelphia: W.B. Saunders, 1975, pp 26-29
3. Newton TH, Potts DG: Radiology of the Skull and Brain. St. Louis: C.V. Mosby, vol 1, book 2, 1971, pp 492-496

Gamut H-14

OPTIC NERVE ENLARGEMENT (ON CT OR MRI)

Neoplastic

COMMON
1. Meningioma of optic nerve sheath, or of intracranial origin
2. Optic nerve glioma

UNCOMMON
1. Hemangioblastoma
2. Lymphoma$_g$, leukemia
3. Metastasis or local extension of ocular tumor (eg, retinoblastoma, melanoma)
4. Neurofibroma

Nonneoplastic

UNCOMMON
1. Central retinal vein occlusion
2. Cyst of optic nerve sheath
3. Dural ectasia
4. Graves' disease (late)
5. Hematoma, traumatic or other

6. Increased intracranial pressure (with papilledema)
7. Multiple sclerosis
8. Optic neuritis
9. Pseudotumor of orbit
10. Sarcoidosis
11. Toxoplasmosis
12. Tuberculosis
13. Vascular lesion (eg, AV malformation—Wyburn-Mason S.; aneurysm of ophthalmic artery; hemangioma; varix, venous occlusion)

References:

1. Azar-Kia B, et al: Optic nerve tumors: Role of magnetic resonance imaging and computed tomography. Radiol Clin North Am 1987;25:561-581
2. Curtin HD: Pseudotumor. Radiol Clin North Am 1987; 25: 583-599
3. Eisenberg RL: Clinical Imaging: An Atlas of Differential Diagnosis. (ed 2) Rockville, MD: Aspen Publ, 1992, pp 962-965
4. Flanders AE, et al: Orbital lymphoma: Role of CT and MRI. Radiol Clin North Am 1987;25:601-613
5. Forbes GS: Computed tomography of the orbit. Radiol Clin North Am 1982;20:37-49
6. Johns TT, Citrin CM, Black J: CT evaluation of perineural orbital lesions: Evaluation of the "tram-track sign. AJNR 1984;5:587-590
7. Leo JS, Halpern J, Sackler JP: Computed tomography in the evaluation of orbital infections. CT 1980;4:133-138
8. Peyster RG, Hoover E: Computed Tomography in Orbital Disease and Neuro-ophthalmology. Chicago: Year Book Medical Publ, 1984
9. Peyster RG, Hoover E, Hershey BL: High resolution CT of lesions of the optic nerve. AJNR 1983;4:169-174
10. Post MJ, Quencer RM, Tabei SZ: CT demonstration of sarcoidosis of the optic nerve, frontal lobes and falx cerebri: Case report and literature review. AJNR 1982;3:523-526
11. Sobel DF, Salvolini U, Newton TH: Ocular and orbital pathology. In: Newton TH, Hasso AN, Dillon WP (eds): Modern Neuroradiology, vol 3. Computed Tomography of the Head and Neck. New York: Raven Press, 1988, pp 9.17-9.24
12. Staubach B: Enlarged optic nerve. Semin Roentgenol 1984;19:83
13. Swenson SA, Forbes GS, Younge BR, et al: Radiologic evaluation of tumors of the optic nerve. AJNR 1982;3:319-326
14. Unsöld R, DeGroot J, Newton TH: Images of the optic nerve: Anatomic-CT correlation. AJNR 1980;1:317-324

Gamut H-15

OPTIC NERVE "TRAM-TRACK" SIGN (DISTINCT OPTIC NERVE WITH PERINEURAL ENHANCEMENT ON CT)

COMMON
1. Optic nerve sheath meningioma

UNCOMMON
1. Carcinomatous infiltration (eg, from lacrimal gland)
2. Erdheim-Chester disease
3. Hemangioma
4. Lymphoma$_g$, leukemia
5. Metastasis
6. Neurofibroma
7. Normal variant
8. Optic neuritis
9. Perioptic hemorrhage
10. Pseudotumor of orbit
11. Retinoblastoma
12. Sarcoidosis

References:
1. Johns TT, Citrin CM, Black J: CT evaluation of perineural orbital lesions: Evaluation of the "tram-track" sign. AJNR 1984;5:587-590
2. Lee SH, Rao K: Cranial Computed Tomography and MRI. (ed 2) New York: McGraw-Hill, 1987, p 148
3. Peyster RG, Hoover E: Computed Tomography in Orbital Disease and Neuro-ophthalmology. Chicago: Year Book Medical Publ, 1984
4. Post MJ, Quencer RM, Tabei SZ: CT demonstration of sarcoidosis of the optic nerve, frontal lobes and falx cerebri: Case report and literature review. AJNR 1982; 3:523-526

Gamut H-16

ENLARGEMENT OF THE RECTUS MUSCLES OF THE EYE (ON CT OR MRI)

COMMON
1. Thyroid ophthalmopathy (Graves' disease)

UNCOMMON
1. Acromegaly
2. Amyloidosis
3. Brown S.
4. Granulomatous disease (eg, tuberculosis, sarcoidosis, Tolosa-Hunt S.)
5. Hemangioma; hemangiopericytoma
6. Increased venous pressure (eg, AV malformation; carotid-cavernous fistula; cavernous sinus thrombosis)
7. Lymphoma$_g$, leukemia, Burkitt's tumor
8. Metastasis (incl. neuroblastoma)
9. Orbital myositis or cellulitis (eg, from adjacent sinusitis)
10. Orbital trauma; foreign body reaction
11. Pseudotumor of orbit
12. Rhabdomyosarcoma; rhabdomyoma
13. Wegener's granulomatosis; lethal midline granuloma

References:
1. Bryan RN, Craig JA: The eye: CT of the orbit. In: Bergeron RT, Osborn AG, Som PM: Head and Neck Imaging Excluding the Brain. St. Louis: C.V. Mosby, 1984, pp 603-606
2. Eisenberg, RL: Clinical Imaging: An Atlas of Differential Diagnosis. (ed 2) Rockville, MD: Aspen Publ, 1992, pp 974-975
3. Peyster RG, Hoover E: Computed Tomography in Orbital Disease and Neuro-ophthalmology. Chicago: Year Book Medical Publ, 1984
4. Sobel DF, Salvolini U, Newton TH: Ocular and orbital pathology. In: Newton TH, Hasso AN, Dillon WP (eds): Modern Neuroradiology, vol 3. Computed Tomography of the Head and Neck. New York: Raven Press, 1988, pp 9.25-9.34

Gamut H-17

UNILATERAL EXOPHTHALMOS (PROPTOSIS)

Systemic Disease

COMMON
1. Hyperthyroidism, thyrotoxicosis

Bone Disease

COMMON
1. Fracture with retro-orbital hematoma or orbital emphysema
2. Metastasis

UNCOMMON
1. Bone neoplasm, benign or malignant (eg, osteosarcoma)
2. Craniosynostosis, severe (See C-1)
3. Fibrous dysplasia, ossifying fibroma
4. Histiocytosis X_g
5. Infantile cortical hyperostosis (Caffey's disease)
6. Myeloma
7. Neurofibromatosis
8. Osteoma of a paranasal sinus
9. Osteomyelitis
10. Osteopetrosis
11. Paget's disease
12. Thalassemia

Paranasal Sinus or Nasopharyngeal Disease with Intraorbital Extension

COMMON
1. Carcinoma, lymphoepithelioma, or other neoplasm
2. Mucocele

UNCOMMON
1. Sinusitis

Primary Orbital Soft Tissue Disease (Including Extension from an Intracranial Lesion)

COMMON
1. Abscess, cellulitis, or myositis (retrobulbar or periorbital)
2. Granuloma
3. Hemangioma, lymphangioma
4. Lacrimal gland tumor
5. Lymphoma$_g$, leukemia, Burkitt's tumor
6. Meningioma (orbital or sphenoid ridge)
7. Metastatic or invasive neoplasm
8. Optic nerve glioma
9. Pseudotumor of orbit
10. Retinoblastoma
11. Spindle cell neoplasm$_g$, benign or malignant (eg, rhabdomyosarcoma)

UNCOMMON
1. Carotid artery aneurysm, carotid-cavernous fistula, cavernous sinus thrombosis, AV malformation (congenital or traumatic)
2. Cholesteatoma, epidermoid
3. Dermoid, teratoma
4. Foreign body
5. Hydatid cyst
6. Neurofibroma, neurilemoma
7. Optic neuritis
8. Orbital meningocele or encephalocele (congenital or traumatic)
9. Orbital varices
10. [Pseudoproptosis (eg, large eye, normal asymmetry)]
11. Retrobulbar infarcts in sickle cell anemia
12. Sympathicoblastoma; neuroblastoma

References:
1. Bullock LJ, Reeves RJ: Unilateral exophthalmos: Roentgenographic aspects. AJR 1959;82:290-299
2. Lee KF, Hodes PJ, Greenberg L, et al: Three rare causes of unilateral exophthalmos. Radiology 1968;90:1009-1015

3. Lloyd GAS: The radiological investigation of proptosis. Br J Radiol 1970;43:1-18
4. Newton TH, Potts DG: Radiology of the Skull and Brain. St. Louis: C.V. Mosby, vol 1, book 2, 1971, pp 468-469
5. Price HI, Danziger A: The computerized tomographic findings in pediatric orbital tumors. Clin Radiol 1979;30:435-440
6. Vade E, Armstrong D: Orbital rhabdomyosarcoma in childhood. Radiol Clin North Am 1987;25:701-714
7. Weber AL, Dallow RL, Momose KJ: Evaluation of orbital and eye lesions by radiographic examination, ultrasound and computerized axial tomography. American Roentgen Ray Society Scientific Exhibit, Atlanta, 1975

Gamut H-18

DEFORMITY AND DIMENSIONAL CHANGES IN THE EYEBALL (ON CT OR MRI)

COMMON

*1. Coloboma of globe
 2. Microphthalmos
*3. Neoplasm (retinal, choroidal, scleral)
 4. Phthisis bulbi
 5. Trauma

UNCOMMON

*1. Axial myopia
*2. Congenital glaucoma (buphthalmos)
*3. Macrophthalmos
*4. Posterior staphyloma
 5. Pseudotumor of orbit
 6. Surgical scleral banding
 7. Wegener's granulomatosis

*May show enlarged eye with increased size of globe.

Reference:

1. Osborne DR: CT Analysis of Deformity and Dimensional Changes in the Eyeball. American Roentgen Ray Society Scientific Exhibit, Boston, 1985

H. Head and Neck

INTRAORBITAL CALCIFICATION
(See Gamuts H-20, H-21)

COMMON
1. Cataract (lens)
2. [Foreign body; fracture fragment]
3. Phlebolith (eg, orbital varices, venous malformation, cavernous hemangioma, AV malformation or shunt)
4. Phthisis bulbi (trauma or infection with shrunken globe)
5. Retinoblastoma

UNCOMMON
1. Aneurysm or atherosclerosis of internal carotid or ophthalmic artery; vascular calcification (eg, diabetes)
2. Collagen disease$_g$ (eg, band keratopathy of cornea in rheumatoid arthritis)
3. Congenital syndromes
   a. Cryptophthalmia S.
   b. Fetal cytomegalovirus infection
   c. Neurofibromatosis
   d. Oculo-dento-osseous dysplasia
   e. von Hippel-Lindau S.
4. Drusen
5. Glaucoma
6. Hematoma; myositis ossificans of extraocular muscles
7. Hypercalcemia (conjunctiva or cornea) (eg, in hyper-vitaminosis D, primary or secondary hyperparathyroidism, metastases, multiple myeloma, milk-alkali S., idiopathic hypercalcemia)
8. Idiopathic
9. Infection, intraocular (eg, abscess, bacterial ophthalmitis, tuberculosis, syphilis)
10. Intraorbital neoplasm (eg, meningioma, hemangioma, dermoid, teratoma, optic glioma, plexiform neurofibroma, choroidal osteoma, hamartoma, lacrimal gland carcinoma, hemangioendothelioma, metastasis)
11. Mucocele invading orbit

12. [Osteoma; fibrous dysplasia]
13. Parasitic disease$_g$ (eg, hydatid cyst, cysticercosis, toxoplasmosis)
14. Phakoma
15. Radiation therapy
16. Retinal disease (eg, detachment, retinitis, fibrosis, retrolental fibroplasia)

References:

1. Ashton N: Calcareous degeneration and ossification. In: Duke-Elder S (ed): System of Ophthalmology. St. Louis: C.V. Mosby, 1962
2. Edwards MK, Buncic JR, Harwood-Nash DC: Optic disk drusen: Case report. JCAT 1982;6:383-384
3. Newton TH, Potts DG: Radiology of the Skull and Brain. St. Louis: C.V. Mosby, vol 1, book 2, 1971, pp 525-540
4. Sundheim JL, Lapayowker MS: Calcification and ossification within the orbit. Radiology 1976;121:391-397

Gamut H-20

GLOBE CALCIFICATION (ON CT)

Neoplasm within the Globe

COMMON
1. Retinoblastoma

UNCOMMON
1. Choroidal osteoma

Neoplasm Infiltrating Posterior Globe from Optic Nerve

COMMON
1. Meningioma of optic nerve sheath

UNCOMMON
1. Hamartoma (tuberous sclerosis)
2. Optic nerve glioma or neurofibroma
3. Sarcoidosis of optic nerve sheath

Trauma

COMMON
1. Phthisis bulbi (result of chronic posttraumatic degeneration or infection)

UNCOMMON
1. Chronic retinal detachment
2. Postoperative

Miscellaneous

COMMON
1. Drusen
2. Lens (senile cataract)

UNCOMMON
1. Hypercalcemic states
2. Radiation therapy
3. Retrolental fibroplasia
4. Toxoplasmosis
5. Vascular lesion (eg, Sturge-Weber S., von Hippel-Lindau S.)

References:
1. Johns TT, Citrin CM, Black J: CT evaluation of perineural orbital lesions: Evaluation of the "tram track" sign. AJNR 1984;5:587-590
2. Peyster RG, Hoover E: Computed Tomography in Orbital Disease and Neuro-Ophthalmology. Chicago: Year Book Med Publ, 1984
3. Sobel DF, Salvolini U, Newton TH: Ocular and orbital pathology. In: Newton TH, Hasso AN, Dillon WP (eds): Modern Neuroradiology, vol 3. Computed Tomography of the Head and Neck. New York: Raven Press, 1988
4. Turner RM, Gutman I, Hilal KS, et al: CT of drusen bodies and other calcific lesions of the optic nerve: Case report and differential diagnosis. AJNR 1983;4:175-178

Gamut H-21

EXTRAGLOBAL CALCIFICATION (ON CT)

COMMON
1. Meningioma of optic nerve sheath
2. Trauma, old
3. Vascular (eg, hemangioma, varices with phleboliths; AV malformation; atherosclerosis)

UNCOMMON
1. Dermoid
2. Hypercalcemic states
3. Lacrimal gland neoplasm
4. Neuroblastoma
5. Neurofibroma
6. Optic glioma
7. [Orbital wall abnormality (eg, fibrous dysplasia, osteosarcoma, metastasis from prostate or breast)]
8. Retinoblastoma (infiltrating)

References:
1. Johns TT, Citrin CM, Black J: CT evaluation of perineural orbital lesions: Evaluation of the "tram-track" sign. AJNR 1984;5:587-590
2. Peyster RG, Hoover E: Computed Tomography in Orbital Disease and Neuro-ophthalmology. Chicago: Year Book Medical Publ, 1984
3. Turner RM, Gutman I, Hilal KS, et al: CT of drusen bodies and other calcific lesions of the optic nerve: Case report and differential diagnosis. AJNR 1983;4:175-178

Gamut H-22

LACRIMAL GLAND ENLARGEMENT

COMMON
1. Benign lymphoid hyperplasia
2. Benign mixed tumor (eg, adenoma)
3. Carcinoma (esp. adenoid cystic carcinoma)
4. Lymphoma$_g$, leukemia

UNCOMMON

1. Amyloidosis
2. Dermoid, epidermoid
3. Inflammation (incl. inflammatory pseudotumor)
   a. Acute dacryoadenitis (usually following a viral infection such as mumps or infectious mononucleosis; also after bacterial or fungal infections)
   b. Chronic dacryoadenitis (eg, sarcoidosis, Sjögren S., Mikulicz S.; rarely tuberculosis, syphilis, leprosy)
4. Metastasis

References:

1. Lee SH, Rao K: Cranial Computed Tomography in Orbital Disease and Neuro-ophthalmology. Chicago: Year Book Medical Publ, 1984, pp 147-150
2. Poyet C: Orbits. In: Ravin CE, Cooper C (eds): Review of Radiology. Philadelphia: W.B. Saunders, 1990, p 132
3. Sobel DF, Salvolini U, Newton TH: Ocular and orbital pathology. In: Newton TH, Hasso AN, Dillon WP (eds): Modern Neuroradiology, vol 3. Computed Tomography of the Head and Neck. New York: Raven Press, 1988, pp 9.34-9.37
4. Stewart WB, Krohel GB, Wright JE: Lacrimal gland and fossa lesions: An approach to diagnosis and management. Ophthalmology 1979;86:886

Gamut H-23

CONGENITAL ABNORMALITIES OF THE TEMPORAL BONE

I. ANOMALIES OF THE SOUND CONDUCTING SYSTEM

1. Stenosis, agenesis, or soft tissue or bony atresia plate of external auditory canal
2. Microtia (deformity of auricle), often with dysplasia of external auditory canal as in:
   a. Mandibular facial dysostosis (eg, Treacher Collins S., Franceschetti S.)
   b. Hypoplastic mandibular condyle and flat temporomandibular fossa

---

3. Atresia or hypoplasia of mastoid air cells
4. Hypoplasia or agenesis of middle ear
5. Anomalies of incus and malleus
6. Abnormalities of labyrinthine window and stapes (eg, congenital fixation of stapes footplate, stapedial otosclerosis)

II. ANOMALIES OF THE FACIAL NERVE
1. Abnormal course, shortening, or ectopia of facial nerve

III. ANOMALIES OF THE INNER EAR
1. Anomaly or defect in otic capsule
   a. Michel deformity (hypoplasia or aplasia of petrous pyramid and inner ear structures)
   b. Mondini deformity (abnormal cochlea)

IV. VESTIBULAR AQUEDUCT AND SEMICIRCULAR CANAL ANOMALIES
1. Dilated shortened aqueduct
2. Hypoplasia or aplasia of vestibule and semicircular canals (eg, Waardenburg S.)

V. ANOMALIES OF THE INTERNAL AUDITORY CANAL
1. Hypoplasia of canal
2. Dilated shortened canal (sometimes with chronic hydrocephalus)

VI. DILATED COCHLEAR AQUEDUCT

VII. CONGENITAL OBLITERATIVE LABYRINTHITIS

VIII. CONGENITAL CEREBROSPINAL FLUID OTORRHEA (DUE TO DEFECT IN INTERNAL AUDITORY CANAL AND STAPES FOOTPLATE)

IX. CONGENITAL VASCULAR ANOMALIES

1. High large jugular fossa and bulb
2. Defect in dome of jugular fossa with herniation of bulb into middle ear simulating glomus tumor
3. Ectopic intratemporal course of internal cartoid artery (lateral position of artery which may lie in middle ear and be associated with persistent stapedial artery and aberrant middle meningeal artery)

References:
1. Unger JM: Handbook of Head and Neck Imaging. New York: Churchill Livingstone, 1987, pp 152-155
2. Valvassori GE, Buckingham RA, Carter BL, Hanafee WN, Mafee MF: Head and Neck Imaging. New York: Thieme Medical Publ, 1988, pp 44-64

Gamut H-24

BONE DISORDER ASSOCIATED WITH OTOSCLEROSIS (ON TOMOGRAPHY OR CT)

COMMON

1. Fibrous dysplasia
2. Osteogenesis imperfecta
3. Paget's disease

UNCOMMON

1. Cleidocranial dysplasia
2. Craniometaphyseal dysplasia
3. Hurler S.
4. Osteopetrosis

Reference:
1. Valvassori GE, Buckingham RA, Carter BL, Hanafee WN, Mafee MF: Head and Neck Imaging. New York: Thieme Medical Publ, 1988, pp 158-172

Gamut H-25

LESION OF THE FACIAL CANAL IN THE TEMPORAL BONE (ON TOMOGRAPHY OR CT)

1. Atresia or hypoplasia of canal
2. Cholesteatoma, congenital or acquired
3. Extratemporal lesion extending into canal (eg, meningioma, parotid tumor)
4. Malignant external otitis (*Pseudomonas*)
5. Neurinoma of facial nerve
6. Posttraumatic or postsurgical injury of facial nerve

Reference:

1. Valvassori GE, Buckingham RA, Carter BL, Hanafee WN, Mafee MF: Head and Neck Imaging. New York: Thieme Medical Publ, 1988

Gamut H-26

EROSION OR DESTRUCTION OF TYMPANIC PORTION OF PETROUS BONE, MIDDLE EAR, OR MASTOID

COMMON

1. Cholesteatoma, acquired or congenital (epidermoid - rare in mastoid)
2. Cholesterol granuloma
3. Chronic otitis media (incus and rarely malleus)
4. Fracture of the temporal bone
5. Mastoiditis, acute or chronic
6. [Postoperative defect, mastoidectomy]

UNCOMMON

1. Bone neoplasm, benign or malignant (eg, hemangioma, embryonal rhabdomyosarcoma)
2. Carcinoma of mastoid, external auditory meatus, or middle ear
3. Ceruminous gland tumor
4. Dermoid cyst
5. Epidural mastoid cyst or pneumatocele
6. Glomus jugulare tumor
7. Granuloma (esp. tuberculosis)
8. Histiocytosis X$_g$
9. Keratosis obturans
10. [Large mastoid air cell]
11. Lymphoma$_g$
12. Malignant necrotizing external otitis (acute osteomyelitis of temporal bone in aged diabetic due to *Pseudomonas aeruginosa*)
13. Metastasis
14. Nasopharyngeal neoplasm (invasive)
15. Neurinoma
16. Postmastoidectomy meningocele or meningoencephalocele

References:
1. DuBoulay GH: Principles of X-ray Diagnosis of the Skull. (ed 2) London: Butterworths, 1980, p 195
2. Duggan CA, Hoffman JC, Brylski JR: The efficacy of angiography in the evaluation of glomus tympanicum tumors. Radiology 1970;97:45-49
3. Livingstone PA: Differential diagnosis of radiolucent lesions of the temporal bone. Radiol Clin North Am 1974; 12:571-583
4. Mendez G Jr, Quencer RM, Post JD, et al: Malignant external otitis: A radiographic-clinical correlation. AJR 1979; 132: 957-961
5. Newton TH, Potts DG: Radiology of the Skull and Brain. St. Louis: C.V. Mosby, vol 1, book 1, 1971, pp 424-442
6. Phelps PD, Lloyd GAS: The radiology of cholesteatoma. Clin Radiol 1980;31:501-512
7. Phelps PD, Lloyd GAS: The radiology of carcinoma of the ear. Br J Radiol 1981;54:103-109
8. Valvassori GE, Buckingham RA, Carter BL, Hanafee WN, Mafee MF: Head and Neck Imaging. New York: Thieme Medical Publ, 1988, pp 74-114

SYNDROMES WITH MASTOID ABNORMALITIES

MASTOIDITIS
1. Gradenigo S.
2. Histiocytosis X_g
3. Hyperimmunoglobulinemia E syndrome (Buckley S. or Job S.)
4. Immotile-cilia S.
5. Wiskott-Aldrich S.

UNDERDEVELOPMENT OF MASTOIDS
1. Cleidocranial dysplasia
2. Cockayne S.
3. Craniodiaphyseal dysplasia
4. Craniometaphyseal dysplasia
5. Endosteal hyperostosis (van Buchem S.)
6. Engelmann's disease (diaphyseal dysplasia)
7. Frontometaphyseal dysplasia
8. Hypothyroidism
9. Mucopolysaccharidoses
10. Osteopathia striata
11. Osteopetrosis
12. Otopalatodigital S.
13. Pyknodysostosis
14. Treacher Collins S.

INCREASED PNEUMATIZATION OF MASTOIDS
1. Acromegaly
2. Adrenogenital S.
3. Dyke-Davidoff-Masson S.
4. Lipoatrophic diabetes (total lipodystrophy)

Reference:
1. Taybi H, Lachman RS: Radiology of Syndromes, Metabolic Disorders, and Skeletal Dysplasias. (ed 3) Chicago: Year Book Medical Publ, 1990, p 841

Gamut H-28

EXTERNAL AUDITORY CANAL TUMOR

COMMON
1. Carcinoma (esp. squamous cell; also basal cell carcinoma, melanoma, metastasis)
2. Exostosis

UNCOMMON
1. Adenomatous tumor (adenoma, pleomorphic adenoma, adenoid cystic carcinoma, adenocarcinoma)
2. Ceruminoma (benign ceruminous adenoma)
3. Cholesteatoma
4. Keratosis obturans; invasive keratitis
5. Osteoma (ivory or cancellous)
6. Skin lesion, benign (eg, lipoma, fibroma, sebaceous cyst)

References:
1. Bergeron RT, Osborn AG, Som PM: Head and Neck Imaging Excluding the Brain. St. Louis: C.V. Mosby, 1984, pp 813-817
2. Powell T, Jenkins JPR: Ear, nose and throat: In: Grainger RG, Allison DJ: Diagnostic Radiology. (ed 2) Edinburgh: Churchill Livingstone, 1992, vol 3, p 2141

Gamut H-29

CALCIFICATION IN EAR CARTILAGE (PINNA)

COMMON
1. Boxing or other trauma
2. Frostbite
3. Gout

UNCOMMON

1. Acromegaly
2. Addison's disease
3. Alkaptonuria (ochronosis)
4. Collagen diseases$_g$
5. Diabetes mellitus
6. Diastrophic dysplasia
7. Familial cold hypersensitivity
8. Hypercalcemia
9. Hypercorticism (Cushing S.)
10. Hyperparathyroidism, primary or secondary
11. Hyperthyroidism
12. Hypoparathyroidism
13. Hypopituitarism (anterior lobe)
14. Idiopathic
15. Inflammatory lesions, infection
16. Polychondritis, relapsing
17. Pseudogout (CPPD crystal deposition disease)
18. Sarcoidosis
19. Senility
20. Syphilitic perichondritis
21. Von Meyenburg's disease (systemic chondromalacia)

References:

1. Gordon DL: Calcification of auricular cartilage. Arch Intern Med 1964;113:23-27
2. Greenfield GB: Radiology of Bone Diseases. (ed 5) Philadelphia: Lippincott, 1990
3. Rubin AB, Chan KF: Case report 109. Pinnal calcification associated with acromegaly. Skeletal Radiol 1980;5:51-52
4. Taybi H, Lachman RS: Radiology of Syndromes, Metabolic Disorders, and Skeletal Dysplasias. (ed 3) Chicago: Year Book Medical Publ, 1990, p 840

H. Head and Neck

Gamut H-30

TEMPOROMANDIBULAR JOINT DISEASE

COMMON
1. Degenerative arthritis
2. Rheumatoid arthritis
3. Temporomandibular joint syndrome (limited excursion of mandibular condyle with displacement of the meniscus, usually anteriorly, occasionally posteriorly, best seen on MRI)

UNCOMMON
1. Adjacent bony disease (eg, Paget's disease, fibrous dysplasia)
2. Ankylosing spondylitis
3. Gout (rare)
4. Iatrogenic (eg, multiple steroid injections)
5. Infectious arthritis
6. Juvenile rheumatoid arthritis
7. Loose body
8. Neoplasm (eg, osteochondroma)
9. Osteochondritis dissecans (avascular necrosis)
10. Pigmented villonodular synovitis
11. Psoriatic arthritis

Reference:
1. Barthelemy CR: The temporomandibular joint. In: Unger JM: Handbook of Head and Neck Imaging. New York: Churchill Livingstone, 1987, pp 189-205

Gamut H-31

DEFORMITY, ASYMMETRY, OR OPACIFICATION OF THE NASAL CAVITY

COMMON
1. Congenital deformity of nasal septum
2. Fracture of nasal plates or septum
3. Mucosal swelling (inflammatory, allergic, traumatic)
4. Pseudopolyp or polyp (incl. allergic polyposis, polypoid rhinosinusitis, cystic fibrosis)
5. Rhinolith, foreign body
6. Turbinate abnormality (eg, enlargement, congenital absence)

UNCOMMON
1. Antrochoanal polyp
2. Benign neoplasm (eg, fibroma, neurofibroma, ossifying fibroma, osteoma)
3. Carcinoma of nose or antrum
4. Choanal atresia or stenosis
5. Dermoid cyst
6. Encephalomeningocele, transsphenoid
7. Esthesioneuroblastoma (olfactory neuroblastoma)
8. Hypoplasia of nasal bones in various congenital syndromes
9. Inverting papilloma
10. Lymphoma$_g$
11. Mucocele
12. Rhinoscleroma with granulomatous mass
13. Wegener's granuloma

References:
1. DuBoulay GH: Principles of X-ray Diagnosis of the Skull. (ed 2) London: Butterworths, 1980
2. Hall RE, Delbalso AM, Carter LC: Radiography of the sinonasal tract. In: Delbalso AM: Maxillofacial Imaging. Philadelphia: W.B. Saunders, 1990, pp 139-207

H. Head and Neck

Gamut H-32

TUMORS AND TUMOR-LIKE LESIONS OF THE NASOPHARYNX, NASAL CAVITY, AND PARANASAL SINUSES

Benign

COMMON
1. Inflammatory polyp; polypoid rhinosinusitis
2. Juvenile angiofibroma
3. [Lymphoid tissue, adenoids]
4. Mucocele
5. Mucous retention cyst
6. Osteoma

UNCOMMON
1. Adenoma
2. Ameloblastoma
3. Amyloidosis
4. Antrochoanal polyp
5. AV fistula
6. Branchial cleft cyst
7. Chondroma
8. Dentigerous (follicular) cyst
9. Dermoid, teratoma
10. Encephalocele, meningocele
11. Epithelial papilloma (inverting and squamous)
12. Fibroma, desmoid tumor
13. Giant cell reparative granuloma
14. Giant cell tumor
15. Granuloma (eg, tuberculosis, sarcoidosis)
16. Hamartoma
17. Hemangioma
18. Histiocytosis X_g
19. Inclusion cyst
20. Lipoma
21. Lymphangioma

22. Nasoalveolar cyst
23. Neurogenic tumor$_g$ (eg, neurinoma of IX, X, or XI nerve)
24. Odontoma
25. [Rhinolith, foreign body]
26. Rhinoscleroma
27. Salivary gland tumor (eg, Warthin's tumor)
28. Tornwaldt's cyst (notochord remnant)

Malignant

COMMON
1. Carcinoma (esp. squamous cell); lymphoepithelioma (incl. Schmincke tumor)
2. Lymphoma$_g$, Burkitt's tumor
3. Metastasis

UNCOMMON
1. Chordoma
2. Esthesioneuroblastoma (olfactory neuroblastoma)
3. Hemangiopericytoma
4. Malignant histiocytoma
5. Melanoma
6. Plasmacytoma (extramedullary), myeloma
7. Salivary gland neoplasm (eg, carcinoma, mixed tumor)
8. Sarcoma (eg, neurosarcoma, rhabdomyosarcoma, spindle cell sarcoma, fibrosarcoma)
9. Wegener's granulomatosis; lethal midline granuloma

Extension of Neoplasm from Intracranial Cavity to Nasopharynx

COMMON
1. Chromophobe adenoma

UNCOMMON
1. Craniopharyngioma
2. Meningioma
3. Neurinoma, neurofibroma
4. Paraganglioma (glomus jugulare, glomus vagale, or carotid body tumor)

References:
1. Hall RE, Delbalso AM, Carter LC: Radiography of the sino-nasal tract. In: Delbalso AM: Maxillofacial Imaging. Philadelphia: W.B. Saunders, 1990, pp 139-207
2. Unger JM: Handbook of Head and Neck Imaging. New York: Churchill Livingstone, 1987, pp 85-91
3. Valvassori GE, Buckingham RA, Carter BL, Hanafee WN, Mafee MF: Head and Neck Imaging. New York: Thieme Medical Publ, 1988, pp 219-234

Gamut H-33

NASOPHARYNGEAL (AND/OR INFRATEMPORAL FOSSA) LESION

COMMON
1. Abscess (retropharyngeal) or cellulitis
2. Cervical spine lesion, including fracture
3. Enlarged adenoids, tonsils
4. Hematoma
5. Juvenile angiofibroma
6. Malignant nasopharyngeal neoplasm (esp. carcinoma, lymphoepithelioma, lymphoma$_g$, rhabdomyosarcoma, plasmacytoma) (See H-32)

UNCOMMON
1. Amyloidosis
2. Aneurysm of internal carotid artery
3. Antrochoanal polyp
4. AV malformation
5. Benign nasopharyngeal neoplasm, other (See H-32)
6. Bone sarcoma (eg, chondrosarcoma, osteosarcoma)
7. Chordoma of clivus
8. Encephalocele, transsphenoid
9. Foreign body
10. Inflammatory polyp; polypoid rhinosinusitis

11. Lymphadenopathy, other (eg, infectious mono-
    nucleosis, sinus histiocytosis)
12. Meningioma of skull base
13. Metastasis
14. Mucocele
15. [Nasal polyp; enlarged turbinate]
16. Neoplasm extending from sphenoid, ethmoid, or
    maxillary sinus, nasal fossa, or parotid gland
17. Rhinoscleroma
18. Sarcoidosis
19. Tornwaldt's cyst (notochord remnant)
20. Tuberculosis of nasopharynx or cervical spine

References:

1. Jing B: Tumors of the nasopharynx. Radiol Clin North Am
   1970;8:323-342
2. Newton TH, Potts DG: Radiology of the Skull and Brain. St.
   Louis: C.V. Mosby, vol 1, book 1, 1971, pp 251-258
3. Swischuk LE: Imaging of the Newborn, Infant, and Young
   Child. (ed 3) Baltimore: Williams & Wilkins, 1989
4. Unger JM: Handbook of Head and Neck Imaging. New York:
   Churchill Livingstone, 1987
5. Valvassori GE, Buckingham RA, Carter BL, Hanafee WN,
   Mafee MF: Head and Neck Imaging. New York: Thieme
   Medical Publ, 1988

Gamut H-34

LESIONS OF THE PTERYGOPALATINE (SPHENOMAXILLARY) FOSSA

COMMON

1. Juvenile angiofibroma
2. Malignant neoplasm, invasive (eg, carcinoma, melanoma, rhabdomyosarcoma, esthesioneuroblastoma)
3. Meningioma of sphenoid wing or nasal fossa
4. Metastasis
5. Trauma with fracture of pterygoid plates (eg,
   zygomatico-maxillary and Le Fort fractures)

UNCOMMON
1. Aneurysm (carotid-cavernous sinus, paraclinoid)
2. Hyperostotic bone disease (eg, fibrous dysplasia, Paget's disease, meningioma, chronic osteomyelitis)
3. Inflammatory disease (eg, necrotizing granuloma, fungal infection, chronic hypertrophic polypoid rhinosinusitis)
4. Inverting papilloma
5. Mucocele (sphenoethmoid)
6. Pituitary adenoma or trigeminal neurinoma extending into base of pterygoid plates
7. Soft tissue tumor extension from parotid gland, nasopharynx, or cervical nodes

Reference:
1. Osborn AG: The pterygopalatine (sphenomaxillary) fossa. In: Bergeron RT, Osborn AG, Som PM: Head and Neck Imaging Excluding the Brain. St. Louis: C.V. Mosby, 1984, pp 172-185

Gamut H-35

ABNORMALITIES OF THE PHARYNX
(See Gamuts H-46 to H-48)

CONGENITAL
1. Choanal atresia
2. Cleft palate
3. Cyst (Tornwaldt's cyst, parapharyngeal cyst)
4. Encephalocele, meningocele

FUNCTIONAL DISORDER
1. Functional nasopharyngeal obstruction by enlarged adenoids or uvula (eg, pickwickian S., hyper-somnolence states)
2. Swallowing disorder (eg, myasthenia gravis, scleroderma, dysautonomia)

TRAUMA

1. Fracture (eg, pterygoid plates, angle of mandible)
2. Puncture wound of nasophyarynx or pharynx (air in soft tissues, abscess, airway distortion)
3. Thorotrast injury to pharyngeal soft tissues and carotid arteries

INFECTION

1. Abscess
2. Adenoid hypertrophy, tonsillitis
3. Fungus disease$_g$ (eg, mucormycosis, actinomycosis, candidiasis)
4. Granulomatous disease (eg, tuberculosis, sarcoidosis, rhinoscleroma)

NEOPLASM (See H-32)

Reference:

1. Valvassori GE, Buckingham RA, Carter BL, Hanafee WN, Mafee MF: Head and Neck Imaging. New York: Thieme Medical Publ, 1988

Gamut H-36

HYPOPLASTIC OR ABSENT PARANASAL SINUSES (USUALLY FRONTAL)

COMMON

1. Congenital absence or hypoplasia
2. Cretinism, hypothyroidism
3. Fibrous dysplasia, leontiasis ossea
4. Kartagener S.
5. Paget's disease
6. Primary anemia$_g$ (esp. thalassemia, sickle cell)
7. Trisomy 21 S. (Down S.)

UNCOMMON

1. Cleidocranial dysplasia
2. Cockayne S.
3. Craniodiaphyseal dysplasia
4. Craniometaphyseal dysplasia
5. Frontometaphyseal dysplasia
6. Hyperphosphatasia
7. Hypopituitarism
8. Maxillonasal dysplasia (Binder S.)
9. Median cleft face S.
10. Metaphyseal chondrodysplasia (Jansen)
11. Osteodysplasty (Melnick-Needles S.)
12. Osteopathia striata with cranial sclerosis
13. Osteopetrosis
14. Otopalatodigital S.
15. Prader-Willi S.
16. Pyknodysostosis
17. Schwarz-Lélek S.
18. Treacher Collins S.

Reference:

1. Taybi H, Lachman RS: Radiology of Syndromes, Metabolic Disorders, and Skeletal Dysplasias. (ed 3) Chicago: Year Book Medical Publ, 1990, p 851

Gamut H-37

OPACIFICATION OF ONE OR MORE PARANASAL SINUSES

COMMON

*1. Hemorrhage or edema from trauma or surgery; epistaxis; barotrauma
2. [Hypoplasia or aplasia of a sinus]
3. Inflammatory mass (eg, nonsecretory cyst, mucous retention cyst, polyp, mucocele, pyocele)
4. Sinusitis

5. [Spurious opacification (eg, swelling of soft tissues of cheek; technical-poor positioning; increased thickness of adjacent bone—fibrous dysplasia, Paget's disease, thalassemia, craniometaphyseal dysplasia)]

UNCOMMON
1. Cystic fibrosis (mucoviscidosis)
*2. Granulomatous or other infectious disease
    a. Fungus disease (eg, mucormycosis, aspergillosis, actinomycosis, blastomycosis, rhinosporidiosis)
    b. Glanders (*Pseudomonas mallei*)
    c. Leprosy
    d. Rhinoscleroma
    e. Sarcoidosis
    f. Syphilis
    g. Tuberculosis
3. Kartagener S; immotile-cilia S. (sinusitis)
*4. Neoplasm, benign or malignant (eg, carcinoma, lymphoma$_g$)
*5. Polypoid rhinosinusitis
*6. Wegener's granulomatosis; lethal midline granuloma

*Often with bone destruction.

Gamut H-38

FLUID LEVEL IN A PARANASAL SINUS

COMMON
1. Fracture of sinus wall with hemorrhage
2. Sinusitis, acute

UNCOMMON
1. Iatrogenic (eg, antral lavage; nasal packing for epistaxis; indwelling nasogastric tube)
2. Neoplasm (eg, osteoma or carcinoma of sinus)
3. Normal (infant)

Reference:
1. Ogawa TK, Bergeron RT, Whitaker CW, et al: Air-fluid levels in the sphenoid sinus in epistaxis and nasal packing. Radiology 1976;118:351-354

Gamut H-39

MASS IN A PARANASAL SINUS

COMMON
*1. Carcinoma (esp. squamous cell; also adenocarcinoma, adenoid cystic; cylindroma)
 2. Encapsulated exudate, pus, or blood
*3. Extrinsic neoplasm invading sinus (eg, pituitary, orbital, oral, or nasopharyngeal; chordoma; juvenile angiofibroma; lymphoepithelioma; Burkitt's tumor)
*4. Fracture with hematoma (eg, blow-out fracture of orbit)
 5. Impacted tooth (maxillary sinus)
 6. Mucocele (esp. frontal or ethmoid)
 7. Mucosal edema or inflammation (eg, from sinusitis due to allergy or infection)
 8. Mucous retention cyst; serous or nonsecretory cyst
*9. Osteoma (esp. frontal or ethmoid)
10. Polyp or pseudopolyp (incl. cystic fibrosis)
*11. [Spurious opacification (eg, swelling of soft tissues of cheek; technical-poor positioning; increased thickness of adjacent bone-fibrous dysplasia, Paget's disease, thalassemia, craniometaphyseal dysplasia)]

UNCOMMON
 1. Antrochoanal polyp (maxillary sinus)
 2. Barotrauma
*3. Benign neoplasm, other (eg, osteochondroma, hemangioma, hemangiopericytoma, dermoid, lipoma, ossifying fibroma, giant cell tumor, aneurysmal bone cyst)
*4. Encephalocele
*5. Epithelial papilloma (squamous and inverting)

*6. Granulomatous disease (eg, tuberculosis, syphilis, leprosy, glanders, fungus disease$_g$, sarcoidosis, rhinoscleroma, giant cell granuloma)
*7. Histocytosis X$_g$
*8. Metastasis (esp. renal, lung, breast)
*9. Myeloma, plasmacytoma (extramedullary)
*10. Neurogenic tumor (eg, schwannoma, neurofibroma, neurocele, meningioma)
*11. Odontogenic cyst or tumor (eg, dentigerous cyst, globulo-maxillary cyst, odontoma) at base of maxillary antrum
*12. Polypoid rhinosinusitis
*13. Surgical ciliated cyst (post-Caldwell-Luc operation)
*14. Wegener's granulomatosis; lethal midline granuloma

*Usually with bone involvement.

Reference:

1. Unger JM: Handbook of Head and Neck Imaging. New York: Churchill Livingstone, 1987

Gamut H-40

SYNDROMES WITH SALIVARY GLAND ABNORMALITY

1. Cystic fibrosis
2. Goldenhar-Gorlin S.
3. Hypoglossia-hypodactylia S.
4. Lacrimo-auriculo-dento-digital S. (LADD S.)
*5. Mikulicz S.
*6. Sjögren S.
7. Treacher Collins S.

*Salivary duct ectasia.

Reference:

1. Taybi H, Lachman RS: Radiology of Syndromes, Metabolic Disorders, and Skeletal Dysplasias. (ed 3) Chicago: Year Book Medical Publ, 1990, p 850

Gamut H-41

SALIVARY GLAND ENLARGEMENT

COMMON

1. Mumps
2. Neoplasm (esp. mixed tumor) (See H-43)
3. Stone in duct (esp. in submandibular gland)
4. Suppurative sialadenitis, acute
5. Trauma with hemorrhage, edema, fistula, or sialocele

UNCOMMON

1. Alcoholism, cirrhosis
2. Allergic or drug reaction (eg, sulfa, iodides)
3. Chronic punctate sialadenitis (benign lympho-epithelial disease, sicca S.)
4. Cyst (eg, dermoid, branchial cleft, mucous retention, ranula)
5. Cystic fibrosis (mucoviscidosis)
6. Granulomatous disease involving parotid gland and lymph nodes (eg, sarcoidosis, tuberculosis, atypical myco-bacteria infection, actinomycosis, cat-scratch fever)
7. Hormonal disturbance (eg, diabetes, hypothyroidism, pregnancy)
8. Idiopathic; lipomatous pseudohypertrophy of parotid
9. Infection, other (eg, acute parotitis, recurrent pyogenic parotitis, sialodochitis)
10. Malnutrition, kwashiorkor
11. [Masseter muscle hypertrophy]
12. Mikulicz S. (bilateral salivary enlargement due to lymphoma$_g$, sarcoidosis, or other disease)
13. Mucocele
14. Radiation therapy
15. Sialodochitis fibrinosa
16. Sjögren S. (associated with rheumatoid arthritis, lupus, or scleroderma)
17. Stricture of duct (See H-42)

References:

1. Kreel L: Outline of Radiology. New York: Appleton-Century-Crofts, 1971, p 91
2. Krolls SO: Salivary gland diseases. J Oral Med 1972;27:96-99

3. Som PM, Sanders DE: The salivary glands. In: Bergeron RJ, Osborn AG, Som PM: Head and Neck Imaging Excluding the Brain. St. Louis: C.V. Mosby, 1984, pp 186-234
4. Valvassori GE, Buckingham RA, Carter BL, Hanafee WN, Mafee MF: Head and Neck Imaging. New York: Thieme Medical Publ, 1988

Gamut H-42

SALIVARY DUCT STRICTURE ON SIALOGRAPHY

1. Carcinoma
2. Congenital
3. Infection, inflammation, scarring
4. Radiation therapy
5. Stone
6. Trauma, including surgical

References:

1. Kreel L: Outline of Radiology. New York: Appleton-Century-Crofts, 1971, p 92
2. Valvassori GE, Buckingham RA, Carter BL, Hanafee WN, Mafee MR: Head and Neck Imaging. New York: Thieme Medical Publ, 1988, p 301

Gamut H-43

SALIVARY GLAND NEOPLASM

BENIGN

*1. Hemangioma, lymphangioma
2. Lipoma
*3. Monomorphic adenoma, esp. Warthin's tumor (papillary adenocystoma lymphomatosum; cystadenolymphoma)
4. Neurinoma, neurofibroma

5. Oncocytoma (oxyphilic adenoma)
*6. Pleomorphic adenoma (mixed tumor)

MALIGNANT

1. Acinic cell tumor
*2. Carcinoma
   a. Adenocarcinoma
 *b. Adenoid cystic (cylindroma)
 *c. Carcinoma in pleomorphic adenoma (malignant mixed tumor)
   d. Epidermoid (squamous cell)
 *e. Mucoepidermoid
   f. Undifferentiated
3. Lymphoma$_g$
4. Metastasis (esp. melanoma, carcinoma of skin)
5. Sarcoma

* Common.

References:

1. Seifert G, Miehlke A, Haubrich J, Chilla R: Diseases of the Salivary Glands. New York: Thieme, 1986, pp 171-318
2. Som PM, Sanders DE: The salivary glands. In: Bergeron RT, Osborn AG, Som PM: Head and Neck Imaging Excluding the Brain. St. Louis: C.V. Mosby, 1984, pp 216-231

Gamut H-44

SOFT TISSUE MASS IN THE NECK

COMMON

1. Abscess
2. Lymphadenopathy, esp. metastatic (See H-44A) or tuberculous (scrofula); also benign lymphoid hyperplasia, acute lymphadenitis, systemic lymph node enlargement
3. Lymphoma$_g$

4. Salivary gland enlargement (eg, mumps, stone in duct, neoplasm)
5. Thyroid adenoma, goiter, cyst, or carcinoma

UNCOMMON
1. Actinomycosis
2. Branchial cleft cyst
3. Cervical aortic arch
4. Cervical thymus gland
5. Chemodectoma (carotid body tumor)
6. Cystic hygroma, lymphangioma
7. Dermoid cyst, teratoma
8. Dilated jugular lymph sac
9. Ectopic salivary gland tissue
10. Ectopic thyroid (eg, sublingual)
11. Epidermoid
12. Hemangioma, AV malformation
13. Hemangiopericytoma
14. Hematoma
15. Laryngocele
16. Lipoma
17. Ludwig's angina
18. Mesenchymal tumor
19. Neurofibroma, neuroblastoma
20. Parathyroid adenoma
21. Sebaceous cyst
22. [Subcutaneous emphysema]
23. Thyroglossal duct cyst
24. Venous thrombosis (eg, jugular)

References:
1. Reede DL, Bergeron RT, Osborn AG: CT of the soft tissues of the neck. In: Bergeron RT, Osborn AG, Som PM: Head and Neck Imaging Excluding the Brain. St. Louis: C.V. Mosby, 1984, pp 491-530
2. Warpeha RL: Masses in the neck. In: Wood NK, Goaz PW: Differential Diagnosis of Oral Lesions. (ed 4) St. Louis: Mosby-Year Book, 1991, pp 616-637

Subgamut H-44A

METASTATIC CERVICAL LYMPHADENOPATHY ON CT OR MRI (LOCATION OF LYMPH NODES AND SUSPECTED PRIMARY SITE OF MALIGNANCY)

UPPER CERVICAL NODES

1. Base of tongue
2. Maxillary or ethmoid sinus
3. Nasopharynx
4. Tonsil

MIDDLE AND LOWER JUGULAR NODES

1. Esophagus
2. Larynx
3. Pharynx
4. Thyroid

MIDLINE OR PARATRACHEAL NODES

1. Larynx
2. Lung
3. Thyroid

SUBMAXILLARY NODES

1. Floor of mouth
2. Tongue

SUPRACLAVICULAR NODES

1. Breast
2. Esophagus
3. Lung
4. Stomach

Reference:
1. Reede DL, Bergeron RT, Osborn AG: CT of the soft tissues of the neck. In: Bergeron RT, Osborn AG, Som PM: Head and Neck Imaging Excluding the Brain. St. Louis: C.V. Mosby, 1984, p 529

Gamut H-45

LARGE TONGUE
(MACROGLOSSIA)

COMMON
1. Amyloidosis
2. Cretinism, hypothyroidism
3. Trisomy 21 S. (Down S.)

UNCOMMON
1. Acromegaly
2. Beckwith-Wiedemann S. (fetal visceromegaly)
3. Cyst (eg, duplication, lingual, thyroglossal duct, dermoid)
4. Glycogen storage disease, type II
5. Infant of diabetic mother
6. Jaw or dental deformity with increased mouth size
7. Kocher-Debré-Sémélaigne S.
8. Lingual thyroid
9. Mucopolysaccharidoses (esp. Hurler S.); GM_1 gangliosidosis
10. Muscular dystrophy, myotonia congenita
11. Neoplasm of tongue (eg, hemangioma, lymphangioma, rhabdomyoma, rhabdomyosarcoma, carcinoma)
12. Robinow S.
13. Trauma

References:
1. Jones KL: Smith's Recognizable Patterns of Human Malformation. (ed 3) Philadelphia: W.B. Saunders, 1988
2. Morfit HM: Lymphangioma of the tongue. Arch Surg 1960; 81:761-767
3. Taybi H, Lachman RS: Radiology of Syndromes, Metabolic Disorders, and Skeletal Dysplasias. (ed 3) Chicago: Year Book Medical Publ, 1990, pp 849-850

Gamut H-46

LESIONS OF THE OROPHARYNX

COMMON
1. Carcinoma of tonsil, soft palate, or base of tongue (esp. squamous cell; rarely lymphoepithelioma or transitional cell)
2. Extension of nasopharyngeal or hypopharyngeal tumor to oropharynx
3. [Normal variant (eg, lingual tonsil hypertrophy; prolapse of mucosa through thyrohyoid membrane mimicking oropharyngeal diverticulum)]
4. Thyroglossal duct cyst
5. Tonsillitis; peritonsillar abscess

UNCOMMON
1. Branchial cleft cyst
2. Cystic hygroma (lymphangioma)
3. Dermoid
4. Lipoma
5. Neurofibroma

Reference:
1. Unger JM: Handbook of Head and Neck Imaging. New York: Churchill Livingstone, 1987, pp 91-99

Gamut H-47

INCREASED RETROPHARYNGEAL (PREVERTEBRAL) SPACE IN AN INFANT OR CHILD

COMMON
1. Enlarged adenoids and lymphoid tissue
2. Hematoma or edema from cervical spine injury or fracture

3. Retropharyngeal abscess or cellulitis (eg, from pyogenic adenitis; perforation of pharynx by foreign body or intubation)
4. Retropharyngeal inflammatory lymphadenopathy (bacterial, viral, tuberculous, histoplasmic)
5. [Technical factors (eg, crying; expiratory film; improper positioning with flexion or obliquity of neck; superimposed ear lobe)]

UNCOMMON

1. Cystic hygroma, lymphangioma
2. Dilated jugular veins and carotid arteries from vein of Galen aneurysm or other large intracranial AV malformation
3. Enteric or duplication cyst
4. Lymphadenopathy, noninflammatory (eg, histiocytosis X_g, leukemia, lymphoma$_g$, sinus histiocytosis)
5. Myxedema (hypothyroidism)
6. Neoplasm (eg, hemangioma, angiofibroma, plexiform neurofibroma, ganglioneuroma, neuroblastoma, teratoma, rhabdomyosarcoma)
7. Retropharyngeal goiter
8. Spinal lesion (eg, osteomyelitis, tuberculosis, metastasis, primary neoplasm)
9. Superior vena cava obstruction with edema
10. Traumatic pseudodiverticulum of pharynx (from finger in infant's mouth during delivery)

References:

1. Grünebaum M, Moskowitz G: The retropharyngeal soft tissues in young infants with hypothyroidism. AJR 1970; 108: 543-545
2. Hayden CK Jr, Swischuk LE: Retropharyngeal edema, airway obstruction, and caval thrombosis. AJR 1982;138:757-758
3. McCook TA, Felman AH: Retropharyngeal masses in infants and young children. Am J Dis Child 1979;133:41-43
4. Swischuk LE: Differential Diagnosis in Pediatric Radiology. Baltimore: Williams & Wilkins, 1984, pp 110-111

Gamut H-48

**INCREASED RETROPHARYNGEAL
(PREVERTEBRAL) SPACE
IN AN ADULT
(See Gamut H-47)**

COMMON
1. Abscess or cellulitis
2. Lymphadenopathy (eg, lymphoma$_g$, tuberculosis)
3. Postcricoid carcinoma
4. Spinal osteophytes, neoplasm, or inflammation
5. Trauma (prevertebral edema or hematoma, spine fracture)

UNCOMMON
1. Chordoma
2. Myxedema
3. Retropharyngeal goiter
4. Zenker's diverticulum

Gamut H-49

**LESIONS OF THE HYPOPHARYNX,
LARYNX, AND UPPER TRACHEA**

COMMON
1. Carcinoma of hypopharynx (esp. in pyriform sinus, posterolateral wall, or postcricoid)
2. Carcinoma of larynx
3. Congenital (eg, tracheoesophageal fistula; atresia; hypoplasia; web; stenosis; laryngomalacia)
4. Epiglottic enlargement (esp. epiglottitis)
5. Foreign body
6. Hemangioma, esp. subglottic in children

7. Infection (eg, *Clostridium tetani*, tuberculosis, fungus disease$_g$ - esp. candidiasis)
8. Juvenile papillomatosis
9. Laryngocele (esp. in glassblowers or musicians, or with chronic coughing)
10. Papilloma, squamous cell (solitary)
11. Retropharygeal abscess
12. Tracheal tumor
13. Trauma (incl. intubation)
14. Vocal cord paralysis (eg, involvement of recurrent laryngeal nerve by malignancy; trauma; congenital)
15. Zenker's diverticulum

UNCOMMON

1. Amyloidosis
2. Benign neoplasm of larynx (eg, chondroma, angiofibroma, fibroma, myoma, lipoma, paraganglioma, neurofibroma)
3. Cyst
4. Metastasis
5. Midline granuloma
6. Sarcoidosis
7. Sarcoma
8. Wegener's granulomatosis

Reference:

1. Unger JM: Handbook of Head and Neck Imaging. New York: Churchill Livingstone, 1987, pp 100-135

Gamut H-50

UPPER AIRWAY OBSTRUCTION IN A CHILD, ACUTE OR CHRONIC
(See Gamuts H-46, H-47, H-49)

Acute

COMMON
1. Abscess (peritonsillar, retropharyngeal, mediastinal)
2. Choanal atresia
3. Croup (laryngotracheobronchitis)
4. Epiglottitis, other epiglottic enlargement
5. Foreign body
6. Laryngeal edema (eg, allergic, anaphylactic, or hereditary angioneurotic edema; inhalation of noxious gases; posttraumatic)
7. Retropharyngeal hemorrhage (eg, bleeding or clotting disorder; hematoma from trauma or neck surgery)

UNCOMMON
1. Diphtheria
2. Laryngeal spasm (eg, tetany)
3. Ludwig's angina

Chronic

COMMON
1. Esophageal atresia; tracheoesophageal fistula
2. Extrinsic mass (eg, neoplasm, thyroid mass, cervical lymphadenopathy, cystic hygroma, thyroglossal duct cyst)
3. Intrinsic tracheal mass
4. Tonsil and adenoid hypertrophy
5. Tracheal stricture or stenosis (traumatic, prolonged intubation, postoperative, inflammatory, burn, congenital)
6. Vascular ring (esp. double aortic arch); innominate artery compression

UNCOMMON
1. Antrochoanal polyp
2. Cyst of epiglottis or aryepiglottic folds
3. Esophageal neoplasm
4. Laryngeal web
5. Macroglossia (eg, myxedema)
6. Micrognathia with glossoptosis (eg, Pierre Robin S., Möbius S.; isolated micrognathia)
7. Nasal angiofibroma
8. Papillomatosis
9. Subglottic hemangioma
10. Tracheomalacia; laryngomalacia
11. Vocal cord lesion (eg, laryngeal polyp, papilloma, or cyst)

References:
1. Dunbar JS: Upper respiratory tract obstruction in infants and children. Caldwell Lecture, 1969. AJR 1970;109:227-246
2. Kushner DC, Clifton Harris GB: Obstructive lesions of the larynx and trachea in infants and children. Radiol Clin North Am 1978;16:181-194
3. Schapiro RL, Evans ET: Surgical disorders causing neonatal respiratory distress. AJR 1972;114:305-321
4. Strife JL: Upper airway and tracheal obstruction in infants and children. Radiol Clin North Am 1988;26:309-322
5. Swischuk LE: Radiology of the Newborn, Infant, and Young Child. Baltimore: Williams & Wilkins, 1989

S

Spine and Its Contents (See Section "M" for MRI Evaluation of Spinal Canal Lesions)

ABNORMAL DENSITY OR DESTRUCTION OF VERTEBRAE

S-31   Increased Band(s) of Density in the Subchondral Zones of Vertebrae (Including Rugger Jersey Spine)

S-32   Bone-In-Bone or Sandwich Vertebra

S-33   Increased Vertical (Pin-Stripe) Trabeculation of One or More Vertebral Bodies

S-34   Focal Area of Sclerosis in a Vertebra

S-35   Dense Sclerotic Vertebra, Solitary or Multiple (Including Ivory Vertebra)

S-36   Spinal Osteopenia (Loss of Density)

S-37   Lytic Lesion of the Spine

S-38   Cyst-like Expansile Lesion of the Body and/or Appendages of a Vertebra

ABNORMAL PEDICLES, FORAMINA, OR NEURAL ARCHES

S-39   Abnormal Size or Shape of a Vertebral Pedicle

S-40   Vertebral Pedicle Erosion or Destruction

S-41   Vertebral Pedicle Sclerosis

S-42   Small or Narrow Intervertebral Foramen

S-43   Enlarged Intervertebral Foramen

S-44   Defective or Destroyed Posterior Neural Arches

S-44A   Spinal Bifida Occulta or Aperta

SACRUM

S-45   Sacral Agenesis or Deformity

S-46   Sacroiliac Joint Disease (Erosion, Widening, Sclerosis and/or Fusion)

S-47   Sacrococcygeal or Presacral Mass (See Gamut S-48)

S-48   Primary Neoplasm of the Sacrum

INTERVERTEBRAL DISKS

S-49   Narrow Disk Spaces

S-50   Wide Disk Spaces

7. Campomelic dysplasia (hypoplastic cervical spine, kyphosis)
8. Cervico-oculo-acoustic S. (cervical segmentation malformation)
9. Chondrodysplasia punctata (Conradi's disease) (kyphoscoliosis, atlanto-axial subluxation)
10. Cockayne S.
11. Dysosteosclerosis (platyspondyly)
12. Dyssegmental dysplasia (short spine, ovoid or misshapen vertebrae)
13. Ehlers-Danlos S. (scoliosis, spondylolisthesis)
14. Enchondromatosis (Ollier's disease) (kyphoscoliosis)
15. Fetal alcohol S.
16. Focal dermal hypoplasia (Goltz S.)
17. Freeman-Sheldon S. (whistling face S.)
18. Geroderma osteodysplastica (platyspondyly)
19. GM_1 gangliosidosis; fucosidosis (platyspondyly)
20. Goldenhar S.
21. Hajdu-Cheney S. (kyphoscoliosis, osteoporosis)
22. Holt-Oram S.
23. Homocystinuria (kyphoscoliosis, osteoporosis, "cod-fish vertebrae")
24. Hyperphosphatasia (scoliosis, biconcave vertebrae)
25. Hypochondroplasia (narrow spinal canal, lordosis, platyspondyly)
26. Idiopathic hypercalcemia (Williams S.) (dense vertebrae, kyphoscoliosis)
27. Incontinentia pigmenti S.
28. Kniest dysplasia (platyspondyly, lordosis, kypho-scoliosis, narrow spinal canal)
29. Larsen S. (cervical kyphosis)
30. Marfan S. (scoliosis, spondylolisthesis)
31. Marshall S. (platyspondyly)
32. Metaphyseal chondrodysplasias (Jansen, McKusick) (atlanto-axial instability)
33. Metaphyseal dysplasia (Pyle's disease) (platyspondyly)
34. Metatropic dysplasia (kyphoscoliosis, platyspondyly, atlanto-axial subluxation)
35. Nail-patella S. (osteo-onychodysplasia) (spina bifida)

36. Narrow lumbar spinal canal S.
37. Oculo-mandibulo-facial S. (Hallermann-Streiff S.) (spina bifida)
38. Oculovertebral S. (hemivertebrae, block vertebrae)
39. Osteochondromuscular dystrophy (Schwartz-Jampel S.) (kyphoscoliosis, platyspondyly)
40. Osteodysplasty (Melnick-Needles S.) (increased vertebral height, anterior concavity)
41. Osteoglophonic dwarfism (platyspondyly, narrow spinal canal)
42. Otopalatodigital S. (posterior spinal defects)
43. Parastremmatic dwarfism (kyphoscoliosis, platyspondyly)
44. Patterson S. (pseudoleprechaunism)
45. Popliteal web S. (spina bifida)
46. Prader-Willi S. (kyphosis)
47. Progeria
48. Radial aplasia-thrombocytopenia S.
49. Rothmund-Thomson S. (flat, elongated vertebrae)
50. Rubinstein-Taybi S.
51. Shawl scrotum S. (hypoplastic C1, subluxation C1-C2)
52. Short rib-polydactyly S. (misshapen, poorly ossified vertebrae, coronal clefts)
53. Smith-McCort S. (platyspondyly)
54. Spondylocostal dysostosis (fused, absent, butterfly, or hemivertebrae; kyphoscoliosis)
55. Spondylo-epi-metaphyseal dysplasia (kyphoscoliosis)
56. Spondyloperipheral dysplasia (platyspondyly)
57. Stickler S. (arthro-ophthalmopathy)
58. Trisomy 13 S.
59. Trisomy 18 S.

References:
1. Felson B, (ed): Dwarfs and other little people. Semin Roentgenol 1973;8:258-259
2. Jones KL: Smith's Recognizable Patterns of Human Malformation. Philadelphia: W.B. Saunders, 1988
3. Kozlowski K, Beighton P: Gamut Index of Skeletal Dysplasias. Berlin: Springer-Verlag, 1984, p 41
4. Taybi H, Lachman RS: Radiology of Syndromes, Metabolic Disorders, and Skeletal Dysplasias. (ed 3) Chicago: Year Book Medical Publ, 1990

Gamut S-2

NONSPINAL CONDITIONS ASSOCIATED WITH VERTEBRAL ANOMALIES

COMMON
1. Cloacal abnormality
2. Congenital heart disease
3. Genitourinary abnormality
4. Neurofibromatosis
5. Sprengel's deformity

UNCOMMON
1. Neurenteric cyst; duplication cyst
2. Venolobar S. (eg, scimitar S., lobar agenesis)

Gamut S-3

KYPHOSIS

COMMON
1. Congenital spinal anomaly (eg, fused vertebrae, hemivertebra, spina bifida with meningocele, bony bar)
2. Congenital syndromes (esp. achondroplasia, chondrodystrophies, storage diseases, neurofibromatosis) (See S-1)
3. Fracture, traumatic or pathologic; dislocation
4. Idiopathic
5. Infection (eg, spinal osteomyelitis or tuberculosis—Pott's disease)
6. Neoplasm of spine, primary or metastatic; multiple myeloma
7. Neuromuscular disorder with hypotonia (eg, cerebral palsy, muscular dystrophy, myasthenia gravis)

8. [Normal in infants (thoracolumbar; C2-3 angulation)]
9. Osteoporosis (esp. senile or postmenopausal)
10. Paget's disease
11. Paralysis (eg, poliomyelitis, paraplegia)
12. Posture, faulty or occupational (upper thoracic, changes with position)
13. Rheumatoid or ankylosing spondylitis
14. Scheuermann's disease (juvenile kyphosis)

UNCOMMON
1. Acromegaly; excessive endocrine growth
2. Charcot spine
3. Cretinism, hypothyroidism
4. Generalized weakness
5. Osteomalacia, rickets
6. Radiation therapy atrophy
7. Syringomyelia

Reference:
1. Schmorl G, Junghanns H: The Human Spine in Health and Disease. (ed 2) New York: Grune and Stratton, 1971, pp 344-362

Gamut S-4

SCOLIOSIS

COMMON
1. Chest wall abnormality (eg, asymmetric chest, congenital rib anomalies, Sprengel's deformity)
2. Congenital spinal anomaly (eg, fusion of posterior elements, unilateral bar, meningomyelocele, segmentation anomaly, wedge vertebra, hemivertebra, Klippel-Feil S.)
3. Congenital syndromes (esp. Marfan S., homocystinuria, osteogenesis imperfecta, storage diseases, neurofibromatosis) (See S-1)

4. Idiopathic
5. Infection (eg, spinal tuberculosis, osteomyelitis)
6. Leg shortening or amputation; pelvic tilt; foot deformity
7. Neoplasm, intraspinal or extraspinal, primary or metastatic; multiple myeloma
8. Neuromuscular disorder with hypotonia (eg, cerebral palsy, muscular dystrophy, Friedreich's ataxia)
9. Osteoporosis
10. Paralysis (eg, poliomyelitis, paraplegia, hemiparesis, hemiplegia)
11. Postoperative (eg, thoracoplasty, pneumonectomy)
12. [Postural-changes with position]
13. Pulmonary or pleural disease, unilateral (eg, fibrosis, fibrothorax, empyema, hypoplastic lung)
14. Spasm (eg, retroperitoneal, psoas, or abdominal abscess, inflammation, or hemorrhage; ureteral or renal calculus)
15. Trauma (fracture, subluxation)

UNCOMMON
1. Congenital heart disease (eg, ASD, tetralogy)
2. Neurenteric cyst, duplication cyst
3. Osteoid osteoma
4. Radiation therapy atrophy
5. Rickets
6. Syringomyelia

Reference:

1. Schmorl G, Junghanns H: The Human Spine in Health and Disease. (ed 2) New York: Grune and Stratton, 1971, pp 364-374

Gamut S-5

PARASPINAL SOFT TISSUE MASS

COMMON
1. Abscess
2. Aortic aneurysm; tortuous aorta
3. [Esophageal dilatation; achalasia]
4. Hematoma, traumatic or spontaneous
5. [Hiatal hernia]
6. Idiopathic; anatomic variant
7. Lymphadenopathy, any cause
8. Lymphoma$_g$, leukemia
9. Metastatic neoplasm
10. Myeloma
11. Neurogenic tumor (neurofibroma, neurilemoma, ganglioneuroma, neuroblastoma); intraspinal tumor of hourglass type
12. [Osteoarthritis (spondylosis deformans); other arthritis with spur formation; DISH; extruded disk]
13. Osteomyelitis of spine with abscess (eg, tuberculous, sarcoid, fungal$_g$, brucella, salmonella, other bacterial); nonspecific spondylitis
14. [Pleural effusion, empyema]
15. [Pneumonia, atelectasis]

UNCOMMON
1. Amyloidosis
2. Bochdalek hernia
3. Bronchogenic cyst
4. Chemodectoma
5. Dilated azygos system (eg, superior or inferior vena cava obstruction); mediastinal varices
6. Eosinophilic granuloma of vertebra
7. Extramedullary hematopoiesis (esp. in thalassemia)
8. Hydatid disease
9. Hydroureter; retrocaval ureter
10. Meningocele, all types
11. [Mesothelioma]

12. Mustard operation for transposition of great vessels
13. Neoplasm of spine, primary (eg, giant cell tumor, chordoma, sarcoma)
14. Neurenteric cyst, duplication cyst
15. Other posterior mediastinal or retroperitoneal neoplasm
16. Paget's disease (uncalcified osteoid)
17. Pancreatic pseudocyst or neoplasm
18. Pheochromocytoma; other adrenal neoplasm
19. Retroperitoneal fibrosis
20. Rhabdomyosarcoma, other soft tissue sarcoma
21. Sequestration, extrapulmonary
22. Splenosis
23. Thoracic kidney

References:
1. Gupta SK, Mohan V: The thoracic paraspinal line: Further significance. Clin Radiol 1979;30:329-335
2. Greenfield GB: Radiology of Bone Diseases. (ed 5) Philadelphia: Lippincott, 1990
3. Polansky SM, Culham JAG: Paraspinal densities developing after repair of transposition of the great arteries. AJR 1980; 134:394-396

Gamut S-6

CERVICAL SPINE INJURIES: MECHANISM OF INJURY

FLEXION
1. Anterior subluxation
2. Bilateral interfacetal dislocation
3. Clay-shoveler's fracture
4. Flexion teardrop fracture
5. Simple wedge fracture

FLEXION-ROTATION
1. Rotatory dislocation with interlocking
2. Unilateral interfacetal dislocation

EXTENSION-ROTATION
1. Pillar fracture

VERTICAL COMPRESSION
1. Bursting fracture
   a. Burst fracture, lower cervical vertebrae
   b. Fracture of occipital condyle
   c. Jefferson fracture of atlas

EXTENSION
1. Extension teardrop fracture
2. Hangman's fracture (deceleration, hyperextension)
3. Hyperextension fracture-dislocation
4. Posterior dislocation of atlas with fractured odontoid
5. Posterior neural arch fracture of atlas

SHEARING
1. Fracture of odontoid process

LATERAL FLEXION

References:
1. Bonakdarpour A: Cervical Spine Trauma. American Roentgen Ray Society Refresher Course, Washington, 1986
2. Harris JH Jr: The Radiology of Acute Cervical Spine Trauma. Baltimore: Williams & Wilkins, 1978
3. Kattan KR: Trauma and No-trauma of the Cervical Spine. Springfield, IL: CC Thomas, 1975

Gamut S-7

CERVICAL SPINE INJURIES: STABILITY

STABLE
1. Anterior subluxation
2. Burst fracture (lower cervical vertebrae)
3. Clay-shoveler's fracture

4. Dens fractures, types I and III
5. Pillar fracture
6. Posterior neural arch fracture of atlas
7. Simple wedge fracture
8. Unilateral interfacetal dislocation

UNSTABLE

1. Bilateral interfacetal dislocation
2. Dens fracture, type II
3. Extension teardrop fracture (stable in flexion, unstable in extension)
4. Flexion teardrop fracture
5. Hangman's fracture
6. Hyperextension fracture-dislocation
7. Jefferson fracture of atlas

References:
1. Bonakdarpour A: Cervical Spine Trauma. American Roentgen Ray Society Refresher Course, Washington, 1986
2. Harris JH Jr: The Radiology of Acute Cervical Spine Trauma. Baltimore: Williams & Wilkins, 1978
3. Kattan KR: Trauma and No-trauma of the Cervical Spine. Springfield, IL: CC Thomas, 1975

Gamut S-8

ATLANTO-AXIAL SUBLUXATION OR INSTABILITY

COMMON

1. Incompetence of transverse atlanto-axial ligament (congenital, traumatic, or hyperemic condition)
2. [Normal widening of C1-dens distance in children (up to 4-5 mm)]
3. Rheumatoid arthritis; juvenile chronic arthritis
4. Trauma (with fracture of odontoid or torn transverse ligaments)

UNCOMMON

1. Absent anterior arch of atlas
2. Absent, hypoplastic, or separate odontoid process (os odontoideum)
3. Ankylosing spondylitis
4. Atlanto-occipital fusion
5. Behcet S.
6. Block vertebra C2-C3
7. Congenital syndromes (esp. Down S., Morquio S.) (See S-8A)
8. Gout
9. Lupus erythematosus; CREST S.
10. Pseudogout
11. Psoriatic arthritis
12. Reiter S.
13. Retropharyngeal or nasopharyngeal infection or abscess (child)
14. Tuberculosis

References:

1. Elliott S: The odontoid process in children—is it hypoplastic? Clin Radiol 1988;39:391-393
2. Kattan KR: Trauma and No-trauma of the Cervical Spine. Springfield, IL: CC Thomas, 1975
3. Koss JC, Dalinka MK: Atlantoaxial subluxation in Behcet's syndrome. AJR 1980;134:392-393
4. Martel W: The occipito-atlanto-axial joints in rheumatoid arthritis and ankylosing spondylitis. Am J Roentgenol, 1961; 86:223-240
5. Swischuk LE: Differential Diagnosis in Pediatric Radiology. Baltimore: Williams & Wilkins, 1984, p 433-434
6. Wortzman G, Dewar FP: Rotary fixation of the atlantoaxial joint: rotational atlantoaxial subluxation. Radiology 1968;90: 479-487

Subgamut S-8A

CONGENITAL SYNDROMES WITH ATLANTO-AXIAL SUBLUXATION OR INSTABILITY*

COMMON
1. Chondrodysplasia punctata (Conradi's disease)
2. Marfan S.
3. Mucopolysaccharidosis (eg, Morquio S.)
4. Trisomy 21 S. (Down S.)

UNCOMMON
1. Aarskog S.
2. Diastrophic dysplasia
3. Dyggve-Melchior-Clausen S.
4. Klippel-Feil S.
5. Metaphyseal chondrodysplasia (McKusick)
6. Metatropic dysplasia
7. Mucolipidosis III
8. Patterson S. (pseudoleprechaunism)
9. Pseudoachondroplasia
10. Spondyloepiphyseal dysplasia
11. Winchester S.

*Congenital laxity of ligaments and associated hypoplasia of dens and C1.

References:
1. Rosenbaum DM, Blumhagen JD, King HA: Atlanto-occipital instability in Down syndrome. AJR 1986;146:1269-1272
2. Taybi H, Lachman RS: Radiology of Syndromes, Metabolic Disorders, and Skeletal Dysplasias. (ed 3) Chicago: Year Book Medical Publ, 1990, p 879

Gamut S-9

ODONTOID (DENS) ABSENCE, HYPOPLASIA, OR FRAGMENTATION

COMMON

1. Craniovertebral anomaly (eg, occipitalization of atlas, atlanto-axial fusion, os odontoideum)
2. Klippel-Feil S.
3. Morquio S.
4. Rheumatoid arthritis; ankylosing spondylitis
5. Trauma
6. Trisomy 21 S. (Down S.)

UNCOMMON

1. Achondroplasia
2. Chondrodysplasia punctata (Conradi's disease)
3. Diastrophic dysplasia
4. Dyggve-Melchior-Clausen S.
5. Kniest dysplasia
6. Metaphyseal chondrodysplasia (McKusick)
7. Metastasis
8. Metatropic dysplasia
9. Mucopolysaccharidoses, other (esp. Hurler S.); mucolipidosis III; fucosidosis
10. Multiple epiphyseal dysplasia (Fairbank)
11. Resorption after cervical spine trauma in infancy
12. Smith-McCort S.
13. Spondylo-epi-metaphyseal dysplasia
14. Spondyloepiphyseal dysplasia congenita
15. Tuberculous spondylitis

References:

1. Elliott S: The odontoid process in children—is it hypoplastic? Clin Radiol 1988; 39:391-393
2. Epstein BS: The Spine. Philadelphia: Lea & Febiger, 1976
3. Garber JN: Abnormalities of the atlas and axis vertebrae—congenital and traumatic. J Bone Joint Surg 1964;46A: 1782-1791
4. Gwinn JL, Smith JL: Acquired and congenital absence of the odontoid process. AJR 1962;88:424-431
5. Kozlowski K, Beighton P: Gamut Index of Skeletal Dysplasias. Berlin: Springer-Verlag, 1984, p 47

6. Schlesinger S: Small or hypoplastic dens. Semin Roentgenol 1986;21:241-242
7. Swischuk LE: Differential Diagnosis in Pediatric Radiology. Baltimore: Williams & Wilkins, 1984, p 433
8. Taybi H, Lachman RS: Radiology of Syndromes, Metabolic Disorders, and Skeletal Dysplasias. (ed 3) Chicago: Year Book Medical Publ, 1990, p 880
9. Wackenheim A: Roentgen Diagnosis of the Craniovertebral Region. Berlin: Springer-Verlag, 1974, pp 363-366

Gamut S-10

CRANIOVERTEBRAL JUNCTION ABNORMALITY

Congenital

BONE ABNORMALITY, ASYMPTOMATIC

1. Asymmetric atlanto-axial joint
2. Asymmetric atlanto-occipital joint
3. Posterior atlas arch defect
4. Rachischisis of C 1
5. Third occipital (tertiary) condyle

BONE ABNORMALITY, SYMPTOM-PRODUCING

1. Atlanto-axial fusion or malsegmentation
2. Atlanto-occipital fusion (occipitalization of atlas); hypoplasia of occipital condyle
3. Basilar invagination (See C-10)
4. Odontoid dysplasia with atlanto-axial dislocation; os odontoideum (separate odontoid); hypoplasia or aplasia of dens
5. Stenosis of foramen magnum

CERVICOMEDULLARY ANOMALY

1. AV malformation
2. Chiari malformations
3. Hydromyelia

Acquired

BONE LESION
1. Fibrous dysplasia
2. Inflammatory disease
3. Neoplasm of skull base (primary or metastatic)
4. Paget's disease
5. Posttraumatic or degenerative lesion

EXTRAMEDULLARY LESION
1. Aneurysm
2. Cyst (eg, arachnoid cyst, epidermoid cyst)
3. Neoplasm (eg, meningioma, neurofibroma, lipoma)

INTRAMEDULLARY LESION
1. Glioma
2. Hemangioblastoma
3. Syringomyelia

Reference:
1. Guinto FC Jr, Kumar R, Mirfakhree M: Radiological Society of North America Scientific Exhibit, Washington, 1984

FUSION OF THE CERVICAL SPINE

COMMON
1. Ankylosing spondylitis
2. Block vertebrae, congenital or acquired (eg, trauma, surgery, tuberculosis or other infection)
3. Juvenile chronic arthritis (Still's disease)
4. Rheumatoid arthritis
5. Synostosing intervertebral osteochondrosis; DISH

UNCOMMON
1. Klippel-Feil S.
2. Myositis (fibrodysplasia) ossificans progressiva
3. Psoriatic arthritis

References:
1. Connor JM, Smith R: The cervical spine in fibrodysplasia ossificans progressiva. Br J Radiol 1982;55:492-496
2. Dihlmann VW, Friedmann G: Die röntgenkriterien der juvenil-rheumatischen zervikalsynostose im erwachsenenalter. Fortschr Röntgenstr 1977;126:536-541

Gamut S-12

VERTEBRAL MALSEGMENTATION (SUPERNUMERARY, ABSENT, PARTIALLY FORMED, OR BLOCK VERTEBRAE)

COMMON
1. Chondrodysplasia punctata (Conradi's disease)
2. Diastematomyelia
3. Isolated anomaly
4. Klippel-Feil S.
5. Meningomyelocele

UNCOMMON
1. Aicardi S.
2. Arteriohepatic S. (Alagille S.)
3. Basal cell nevus S. (Gorlin S.)
4. Cat's cry S. (cri du chat S.)
5. Caudal dysplasia S.
6. Cervico-oculo-acoustic S. (Wildervanck S.)
7. Dyssegmental dysplasia
8. Femoral hypoplasia-unusual facies S.
9. Fetal alcohol S.
10. Focal dermal hypoplasia (Goltz S.)
11. Goldenhar S.

12. Holt-Oram S.
13. Incontinentia pigmenti
14. Larsen S.
15. LEOPARD S.
16. Multiple pterygium S.
17. MURCS association
18. Noonan S.
19. Poland S.
20. Robinow S.
21. Split notochord S.
22. Spondylocostal dysostosis
23. Tethered cord S.
24. Trisomy 8 S.
25. Trisomy 18 S.
26. VATER association

References:
1. Kozlowski K, Beighton P: Gamut Index of Skeletal Dysplasias. Berlin: Springer-Verlag, 1984, p 45
2. Taybi H, Lachman RS: Radiology of Syndromes, Metabolic Disorders, and Skeletal Dysplasias. (ed 3) Chicago: Year Book Medical Publ, 1990, p 881

Gamut S-13
CORONAL CLEFT VERTEBRAE

COMMON
1. Chondrodysplasia punctata (Conradi's disease)
2. Kniest dysplasia
3. Metatropic dysplasia
4. Normal variant (esp. in lower thoracic–upper lumbar spine of premature male infant)

UNCOMMON
1. Atelosteogenesis
2. Dyssegmental dysplasia
3. Fibrochondrogenesis

4. Humerospinal dysostosis
5. Malsegmentation of spine
6. Micrognathic dwarfism (Weissenbacher-Zweymuller S.)
7. Trisomy 13 S.

References:
1. Fielden P, Russell JGB: Coronally cleft vertebra. Clin Radiol 1970;21:327-328
2. Kozlowski K, Beighton P: Gamut Index of Skeletal Dysplasias. Berlin: Springer-Verlag, 1984, p 46
3. Rowley KA: Coronal cleft vertebra. J Fac Radiol 1955; 6:267-274
4. Swischuk LE: Differential Diagnosis in Pediatric Radiology. Baltimore: Williams & Wilkins, 1984, pp 398-399
5. Taybi H, Lachman RS: Radiology of Syndromes, Metabolic Disorders, and Skeletal Dysplasias. (ed 3) Chicago: Year Book Medical Publ, 1990, p 880
6. Wollin DG, Elliott GB: Coronal cleft vertebrae and persistent notochordal derivatives of infancy. J Can Assoc Radiol 1961; 12:78-81

Gamut S-14

PROMINENT ANTERIOR CANAL (CENTRAL VEIN GROOVE) OF A VERTEBRAL BODY

COMMON
1. Hypothyroidism
2. Normal (up to age 7)
3. Sickle cell anemia$_g$

UNCOMMON
1. Gaucher's disease
2. Leukemia, lymphoma$_g$
3. Metastatic neuroblastoma
4. Osteopetrosis
5. Progeria
6. Thalassemia major

References:
1. Greenfield GB: Radiology of Bone Diseases. (ed 5) Philadelphia: Lippincott, 1990
2. Mandell GA, Kricum ME: Exaggerated anterior vertebral notching. Radiology 1979;131:367-369
3. Swischuk LE: Differential Diagnosis in Pediatric Radiology. Baltimore: Williams & Wilkins, 1984, pp 399-400

Gamut S-15

CONGENITAL PLATYSPONDYLY

COMMON
1. Hypothyroidism, juvenile; cretinism
2. Morquio S.
3. Osteogenesis imperfecta congenita
4. Spondyloepiphyseal dysplasia, all forms
5. Thanatophoric dysplasia

UNCOMMON
1. Achondrogenesis
2. Achondroplasia (homozygous)
3. Cephaloskeletal dysplasia (Taybi-Linder S.)
4. Diastrophic dysplasia
5. Dyggve-Melchior-Clausen S.
6. Dysosteosclerosis
7. Ehlers-Danlos S.
8. Geroderma osteodysplastica
9. GM_1 gangliosidosis; fucosidosis
10. Homocystinuria
11. Hyperphosphatasia
12. Hypochondroplasia
13. Hypophosphatasia, severe
14. [Idiopathic juvenile osteoporosis]
15. Kniest dysplasia
16. Larsen S.
17. Marshall S.
18. Metatropic dysplasia

19. Oculo-mandibulo-facial S. (Hallermann-Streiff S.)
20. Osteochondromuscular dystrophy (Schwartz-Jampel S.)
21. Osteoglophonic dwarfism
22. Parastremmatic dwarfism
23. Pseudoachondroplasia
24. Rothmund-Thomson S.
25. Short rib–polydactyly S., type 1 (Saldino-Noonan)
26. Smith-McCort S.
27. Spondylo-epi-metaphyseal dysplasia
28. Spondylometaphyseal dysplasia (Kozlowski)
29. Spondyloperipheral dysplasia

References:

1. Kozlowski K; Platyspondyly in childhood. Pediatr Radiol 1974;2:81-88
2. Kozlowski K, Beighton P: Gamut Index of Skeletal Dysplasias. Berlin: Springer-Verlag, 1984, p 43
3. Swischuk LE: Differential Diagnosis in Pediatric Radiology. Baltimore: Williams & Wilkins, 1984, pp 403-404
4. Taybi H, Lachman RS: Radiology of Syndromes, Metabolic Disorders, and Skeletal Dysplasias. (ed 3) Chicago: Year Book Medical Publ, 1990, p 880

Gamut S-16

ANISOSPONDYLY*

1. Campomelic dysplasia
2. Homocystinuria
3. Kniest dysplasia
4. Osteogenesis imperfecta
5. Spondylo-epi-metaphyseal dysplasia
6. Spondyloepiphyseal dysplasia
7. Spondylometaphyseal dysplasia
8. Stickler S. (arthro-ophthalmopathy)

* Irregular flattening of two or more vertebral bodies in the presence of other normal vertebrae.

Reference:

1. Kozlowski K, Beighton P: Gamut Index of Skeletal Dysplasias. Berlin: Springer-Verlag, 1984, p 44

Gamut S-17

SOLITARY COLLAPSED VERTEBRA (INCLUDING VERTEBRA PLANA) (See Gamut S-18)

COMMON
*1. Eosinophilic granuloma (histiocytosis X_g)
*2. Fracture, traumatic or pathologic
*3. Hemangioma
 4. Hyperparathyroidism, brown tumor
*5. Lymphoma$_g$, leukemia,
*6. Metastasis (incl. neuroblastoma)
 7. Myeloma, plasmacytoma
 8. [Normal developmental variant (eg, C5 or C6 or a thoracic vertebra reduced in height)]
 9. Osteomyelitis (eg, tuberculous, fungal$_g$, pyogenic, brucellar, typhoid, syphilitic)
 10. Osteoporosis (eg, senile, postmenopausal)
*11. Paget's disease
 12. Steroid therapy; Cushing S.

UNCOMMMON
 1. Amyloidosis
 2. Benign bone tumor, other (eg, giant cell tumor, aneurysmal bone cyst)
 3. Chordoma
 4. Hydatid disease
 5. Neuropathy (eg, diabetes, syphilis, congenital indifference to pain)
 6. Osteomalacia
 7. Sarcoidosis
 8. Sarcoma (eg, Ewing's, osteosarcoma, chondrosarcoma)
 9. Scheuermann's disease
*10. Traumatic ischemic necrosis (eg, Kümmell's disease)

*May produce vertebra plana.

Gamut S-18

MULTIPLE COLLAPSED VERTEBRAE
(See Gamut S-15)

COMMON

1. Fractures, traumatic or pathologic
2. Hyperparathyroidism, primary or secondary
3. Metastases
4. Multiple myeloma
5. Neuropathy (eg, diabetes, syphilis, congenital indifference to pain)
6. Osteomalacia
7. Osteomyelitis (eg, tuberculous, fungal$_g$, pyogenic, brucellar, syphilitic)
8. Osteoporosis (eg, senile, postmenopausal, idiopathic juvenile; hypogonadism; prolonged immobilization)
9. Scheuermann's disease
10. Sickle cell anemia, other anemias$_g$
11. Steroid therapy; Cushing S.

UNCOMMON

1. Amyloidosis
2. Congenital fibromatosis
3. Convulsions (eg, tetanus, tetany, hypoglycemia, shock therapy)
4. Gaucher's disease
5. Hemangiomatosis (vanishing bone disease)
6. Histiocytosis X$_g$
7. Hydatid disease
8. Hyperphosphatasia
9. Hypophosphatasia
10. Lymphoma$_g$, leukemia
11. Osteogenesis imperfecta
12. Osteolysis (Hajdu-Cheney S.)
13. Paget's disease
14. [Platyspondyly, esp. dwarf syndromes (eg, Morquio S., spondyloepiphyseal dysplasia, pseudoachondro-plasia, thanatophoric dysplasia) (See S-15)]

15. Radiation therapy
16. Rheumatoid arthritis

BICONCAVE ("FISH") VERTEBRAE (INCLUDING STEP-LIKE VERTEBRAE)

COMMON
1. Metastatic disease
2. Osteomalacia, rickets
3. Osteoporosis (eg, senile, postmenopausal, malnutrition, steroid therapy, hyperparathyroidism)
*4. Renal osteodystrophy
*5. Schmorl's nodes
*6. Sickle cell anemia

UNCOMMON
*1. Gaucher's disease
*2. Homocystinuria
3. Lymphoma$_g$
4. Osteogenesis imperfecta
*5. Other anemias$_g$ (eg, thalassemia major, hereditary spherocytosis, iron deficiency)

*"Step-like" vertebra with H-shaped or Lincoln log configuration may occur.

References:
1. Greenfield GB: Radiology of Bone Diseases. (ed 5) Philadelphia: Lippincott, 1990
2. Rohlfing BM: Vertebral end-plate depression: Report of two patients without hemoglobinopathy. AJR 1977;128:599-600
3. Schwartz AM, Homer MJ, McCauley RGK: Step-off vertebral body: Gaucher's disease versus sickle cell hemoglobinopathy. AJR 1979;132:81-85
4. Swischuk LE: Differential Diagnosis in Pediatric Radiology. Baltimore: Williams & Wilkins, 1984, pp 407-408

5. Westerman MP, Greenfield GB, Wong PWK: "Fish vertebrae," homocystinuria, and sickle cell anemia. JAMA 1974; 230:261-262
6. Ziter FMH Jr: Central vertebral end-plate depression in chronic renal disease: Report of two cases. AJR 1979; 132: 809-811

Gamut S-20

WEDGED VERTEBRAE*

1. Chronic hyperflexion of spine; muscular hypotonia
2. Congenital syndromes with thoracolumbar wedging (eg, achondroplasia, hypothyroidism, mucopolysaccharidoses)
3. Hemivertebra
4. Kyphosis (See S-3)
5. Normal variant (minimal wedging in thoracic spine)
6. Pathological fracture in weakened vertebra (eg, metastasis, myeloma, primary neoplasm)
7. Rotoscoliosis (lateral wedging)
8. Scheuermann's disease
9. Trauma (compression fracture)
10. Tuberculosis (gibbus); other chronic infection of spine

*Primarily anterior wedging unless otherwise indicated.

Reference:

1. Swischuk LE: Differential Diagnosis in Pediatric Radiology. Baltimore: Williams & Wilkins, 1984, p 411

Gamut S-21

BEAKED OR HOOK-SHAPED VERTEBRAE IN A CHILD

COMMON
1. Achondroplasia (central anterior wedging)
2. Cretinism, hypothyroidism (inferior beak)
3. Mucopolysaccharidoses (esp. Morquio S.–central beak, Hunter S.–inferior beak, Hurler S.)
4. Neuromuscular disease with generalized hypotonia (eg, Werdnig-Hoffmann disease, Niemann-Pick disease, phenylketonuria, mental retardation)
5. Normal variant in infants (thoracolumbar junction, C2-3 angulation)
6. Scheuermann's disease
7. Trauma, acute or chronic; battered child S. (hyperflexion-compression spinal injury)

UNCOMMON
1. Diastrophic dysplasia
2. Dyggve-Melchior-Clausen S.
3. Immunodeficiency (severe combined) and adenosine deaminase deficiency
4. Marshall S.
5. Mucolipidoses; fucosidosis; mannosidosis
6. Neurofibromatosis (dysplastic vertebrae)
7. Pseudoachondroplasia
8. Spondyloepiphyseal dysplasia
9. Trisomy 21 S. (Down S.)

References:
1. Swischuk LE: The beaked, notched, or hooked vertebra; its significance in infants and young children. Radiology 1970; 95:661-664
2. Swischuk LE: Differential Diagnosis in Pediatric Radiology. Baltimore: Williams & Wilkins, 1984, pp 412-413
3. Taybi H, Lachman RS: Radiology of Syndromes, Metabolic Disorders, and Skeletal Dysplasias. (ed 3) Chicago: Year Book Medical Publ, 1990, pp 879-880

Gamut S-22

CUBOID VERTEBRAE

COMMON
1. Achondroplasia
2. Normal variant (cervical spine and thoracolumbar junction)

UNCOMMON
1. Diastrophic dysplasia
2. Hypochondroplasia
3. Mucopolysaccharidoses
4. Short-rib polydactyly syndromes (eg, Saldino-Noonan S., Majewski S.)
5. Thanatophoric dysplasia

Reference:
1. Swischuk LE: Differential Diagnosis in Pediatric Radiology. Baltimore: Williams & Wilkins, 1984, p 406

Gamut S-23

ROUND VERTEBRAE

COMMON
1. Hypothyroidism, untreated
2. Normal in neonate (esp. thoracolumbar junction) or child with delayed appearance of ring epiphyses
3. Vertebral body underdevelopment (eg, meningo-myelocele)

UNCOMMON
1. Bone dysplasias with "pear shaped" vertebrae (eg, Morquio S.; spondyloepiphyseal dysplasia; Dyggve-Melchior-Clausen S.)

2. Short rib-polydactyly syndromes (eg, Saldino-Noonan S.; Majewski S.)

Reference:
1. Swischuk LE: Differential Diagnosis in Pediatric Radiology. Baltimore: Williams & Wilkins, 1984, pp 409-410

Gamut S-24

TALL VERTEBRAE

COMMON
1. [Block vertebra]
2. Hypotonia (eg, neuromuscular disorders, mental retardation); non–weight bearing
3. Rubella S.
4. Trisomy 21 S. (Down S.)

UNCOMMON
1. Freeman-Sheldon S. (whistling face S.)
2. Marfan S., arachnodactyly
3. Osteodysplasty (Melnick-Needles S.)
4. Proteus S.
5. Spondylocostal dysplasia

References:
1. Gooding CA, Neuhauser EBD: Growth and development of the vertebral bodies in the presence and absence of normal stress. AJR 1965;93:388-393
2. Kozlowski K, Beighton P: Gamut Index of Skeletal Dysplasias. Berlin: Springer-Verlag, 1984, p 44
3. Swischuk LE: Differential Diagnosis in Pediatric Radiology. Baltimore: Williams & Wilkins, 1984, p 408
4. Taybi H, Lachman RS: Radiology of Syndromes, Metabolic Disorders, and Skeletal Dysplasias. (ed 3) Chicago: Year Book Medical Publ, 1990, p 881

FUSED OR BLOCK VERTEBRAE

Congenital

1. Focal dermal hypoplasia (Goltz S.) (anterior fusion)
2. Isolated anomaly (esp. C2-3)
3. Klippel-Feil S.
4. With spinal dysraphism

Acquired

1. Ankylosing spondylitis
2. Infection (esp. tuberculosis)
3. Rheumatoid arthritis (esp. juvenile)
4. Scheuermann's disease
5. Surgical fusion
6. Trauma, severe

Reference:

1. Swischuk LE: Differential Diagnosis in Pediatric Radiology. Baltimore: Williams & Wilkins, 1984, pp 415-416

Gamut S-26

ENLARGEMENT OF ONE OR MORE VERTEBRAE

COMMON
1. Acromegaly; gigantism
2. Paget's disease

UNCOMMON
1. Benign bone tumor (eg, giant cell tumor, hemangioma, aneurysmal bone cyst, osteoblastoma)

2. Compensatory enlargement from non–weight bearing (eg, paralysis)
3. Congenital (eg, block vertebra)
4. Fibrous dysplasia
5. Hydatid disease
6. Hyperphosphatasia

References:
1. Epstein BS: The Spine. (ed 4) Philadelphia: Lea & Febiger, 1976
2. Greenfield GB: Radiology of Bone Diseases. (ed 5) Philadelphia: Lippincott, 1990

Gamut S-27

"SQUARING" OF ONE OR MORE VERTEBRAL BODIES

COMMON
1. Ankylosing spondylitis
2. Paget's disease

UNCOMMON
1. Normal variant
2. Psoriatic arthritis
3. Reiter S.
4. Rheumatoid arthritis

Reference:
1. Jacobson HG: Personal communication

SPOOL-SHAPED VERTEBRAE (ANTERIOR AND POSTERIOR SCALLOPING)

COMMON
1. Hypotonia
2. Neurofibromatosis
3. Normal (occasionally mild in lumbar spine)

UNCOMMON
1. Mucopolysaccharidoses
2. Osteodysplasty (Melnick-Needles S.)
3. Trisomy 21 S. (Down S.); other trisomies

Reference:
1. Swischuk LE: Differential Diagnosis in Pediatric Radiology. Baltimore: Williams & Wilkins, 1984, p 414

ANTERIOR GOUGE DEFECT (SCALLOPING) OF ONE OR MORE VERTEBRAL BODIES

COMMON
1. Aneurysm of aorta
2. Lymphoma$_g$, chronic leukemia
3. Lymphadenopathy from metastases or inflammation
4. Normal variant (lower thoracic, upper lumbar)
5. Tuberculosis

UNCOMMON
1. Adjacent intra-abdominal neoplasm or cyst
2. Cockayne S.
3. Glycogen storage disease

4. Neurofibromatosis (dysplastic vertebra)
5. Osteodysplasty (Melnick-Needles S.)
6. Trisomy 21 S. (Down S.)

Reference:
1. Swischuk LE: Differential Diagnosis in Pediatric Radiology. Baltimore: Williams & Wilkins, 1984, pp 401-402

Gamut S-30

EXAGGERATED CONCAVITY (SCALLOPING) OF THE POSTERIOR SURFACE OF ONE OR MORE VERTEBRAL BODIES

COMMON
1. Achondroplasia
2. Increased intraspinal pressure
3. Neoplasm of spinal canal (eg, ependymoma, dermoid, lipoma, neurofibroma, meningioma)
4. Neurofibromatosis with or without neurofibroma ("dural ectasia"); congenital expansion of the subarachnoid space ("intraspinal meningocele")
5. Normal variant (physiologic scalloping—esp. L4, L5)

UNCOMMON
1. Acromegaly
2. Communicating hydrocephalus, severe
3. Cyst of spinal canal
4. Hydatid disease
5. Other congenital syndromes
   a. Cockayne S.
   b. Diastrophic dysplasia
   c. Dyggve-Melchior-Clausen S.
   d. Ehlers-Danlos S. (dural ectasia)
   e. Marfan S. (dural ectasia)
   f. Metatropic dysplasia

   g. Mucopolysaccharidoses
     (eg, Hurler, Hunter, Morquio)
   h. Osteogenesis imperfecta tarda
   i. Smith-McCort S.
   j. Thanatophoric dysplasia
6. Spinal dysraphism, meningomyelocele
7. Syringomyelia, hydromyelia

References:
1. Greenfield GB: Radiology of Bone Diseases. (ed 5) Philadelphia: Lippincott, 1990
2. Heard G, Payne EE: Scalloping of the vertebral bodies in von Recklinghausen's disease of the nervous system (neurofibromatosis). J Neurol Neurosurg Psychiatry 1962;25: 345-351
3. Howieson J, Norrell HA, Wilson CB: Expansion of the subarachnoid space in the lumbosacral region. Radiology 1968; 90:488-492
4. Kozlowski K, Beighton P: Gamut Index of Skeletal Dysplasias. Berlin: Springer-Verlag, 1984, p 46
5. Leeds NE, Jacobson HG: Plain film examination of the spinal canal. Semin Roentgenol 1972;7:179-196
6. Mitchell GE, Lourie H, Berne AS: The various causes of scalloped vertebrae with notes on their pathogenesis. Radiology 1967;89:67-74
7. Salerno NR, Edeiken J: Vertebral scalloping in neurofibromatosis. Radiology 1970;97:509-510
8. Swischuk LE: Differential Diagnosis in Pediatric Radiology. Baltimore: Williams & Wilkins, 1984, pp 401-402

Gamut S-31

INCREASED BAND(S) OF DENSITY IN THE SUBCHONDRAL ZONES OF VERTEBRAE (INCLUDING RUGGER JERSEY SPINE)

COMMON
1. Compression fracture
2. Hypercorticism, Cushing S., steroid therapy

*3. Hyperparathyroidism, primary or esp. secondary (renal osteodystrophy)
*4. Osteopetrosis
 5. Paget's disease
 6. Sclerosing spondylosis in the elderly

UNCOMMON
 1. Growth arrest lines
 2. Heavy metals (eg, thorotrast, lead)
 3. Hypoparathyroidism, pseudohypoparathyroidism
*4. Idiopathic hypercalcemia (Williams S.)
 5. Leukemia, treated
*6. Myeloid metaplasia (myelosclerosis)
 7. Radiation therapy

*May have the appearance of a "rugger jersey."

Gamut S-32

BONE-IN-BONE OR SANDWICH VERTEBRA

COMMON
 1. Osteopetrosis
 2. Paget's disease
 3. Physiologic in newborn
 4. Renal osteodystrophy, healing

UNCOMMON
 1. Chronic illness (growth arrest lines)
 2. Hypercalcemia; hypervitaminosis D
 3. Lead poisoning, chronic
 4. Radiation therapy
 5. Thorotrast

Reference:
1. Swischuk LE: Differential Diagnosis in Pediatric Radiology. Baltimore: Williams & Wilkins, 1984, p 391

---

4. Idiopathic hypercalcemia (Williams S.)
5. Mastocytosis
6. Multiple myeloma (rare)
7. Osteoblastoma
8. Osteoma, enostoma, bone island
*9. Osteopetrosis
10. Radiation therapy; radium poisoning
11. Rickets, healing
12. Sarcoidosis
13. Sarcoma (eg, osteosarcoma; chondrosarcoma; Ewing's sarcoma)
14. Sickle cell anemia$_g$
15. Spondylosis, chronic sclerosing; intervertebral disc disease
16. Tuberous sclerosis

*Can cause "ivory" vertebra(e).

Reference:

1. Jacobson HG, Siegelman SS: Some miscellaneous solitary bone lesions. Semin Roentgenol 1966;1:314-335

Gamut S-36

SPINAL OSTEOPENIA (LOSS OF DENSITY)

COMMON
1. Anemia$_g$ (esp. sickle cell anemia, thalassemia)
2. Carcinomatosis
3. Hyperparathyroidism, primary or secondary (renal osteodystrophy)
4. Multiple myeloma
5. Osteomalacia
6. Osteoporosis (esp. senile or postmenopausal; prolonged immobilization)
7. Steroid therapy; Cushing S.

UNCOMMON
1. Acromegaly
2. Amyloidosis
3. Fibrogenesis imperfecta ossium
4. Gaucher's disease; Niemann-Pick disease
5. Homocystinuria
6. Hyperthyroidism
7. Hypogonadism (eg, Fröhlich's S.; Turner S.)
8. Leukemia, lymphoma$_g$
9. Osteogenesis imperfecta

Reference:
1. Greenfield GB: Radiology of Bone Diseases. (ed 5) Philadelphia: Lippincott, 1990

Gamut S-37

LYTIC LESION OF THE SPINE

COMMON
1. Hemangioma
2. Histiocytosis X$_g$ (esp. eosinophilic granuloma)
3. Metastasis (incl. neuroblastoma)
4. Myeloma, plasmacytoma
5. Osteomyelitis, spondylitis (eg, tuberculous, sarcoid, fungal, brucellar, other bacterial)
6. Paget's disease
7. Rheumatoid arthritis
8. [Schmorl's nodes]

UNCOMMON
1. Aneurysmal bone cyst
2. Brown tumor of hyperparathyroidism
3. Chondroid lesion
4. Chordoma, notochordal remnant
5. Fibrous dysplasia
6. Giant cell tumor

---

7. Gout
8. Hemangiopericytoma
9. Hydatid disease
10. Intraspinal neoplasm with erosion of vertebra (eg, neurofibroma, meningioma)
11. Lymphoma$_g$
12. [Meningocele, diastematomyelia]
13. Nonossifying fibroma
14. Osteoblastoma
15. Sarcoma (eg, Ewing's, osteolytic osteosarcoma, chondrosarcoma, fibrosarcoma, malignant fibrous histiocytoma, rhabdomyosarcoma)
16. Traumatic ischemic necrosis (Kümmell's disease)

Gamut S-38

CYST-LIKE EXPANSILE LESION OF THE BODY AND/OR APPENDAGES OF A VERTEBRA

COMMON
1. Aneurysmal bone cyst
2. Hemangioma
3. Osteoblastoma

UNCOMMON
1. Chondroid lesion
2. Fibrous dysplasia
3. Giant cell tumor
4. Gout
5. Hemangiopericytoma
6. Hydatid cyst
7. Metastasis
8. Myeloma, plasmacytoma

Gamut S-39

ABNORMAL SIZE OR SHAPE OF A VERTEBRAL PEDICLE

ABSENT OR HYPOPLASTIC PEDICLE
1. Congenital absence or hypoplasia
2. Destroyed pedicle (See S-40)
3. Mucopolysaccharidoses (esp. Hunter S.)
4. Neurofibromatosis
5. [Poorly visualized pedicles C2-C5]
6. Radiation therapy

ENLARGED PEDICLE
1. Compensatory hypertrophy with contralateral deficiency of neural arch
2. Neoplasm (eg, osteoblastoma, hemangioma)

DYSPLASTIC PEDICLE
1. Diastematomyelia
2. Klippel-Feil S.
3. Meningomyelocele
4. Neurofibromatosis
5. Other congenital anomaly

FLATTENED PEDICLE
1. Intraspinal expanding neoplasm or cyst; AV malformation
2. Normal (eg, upper lumbar spine)
3. Syringomyelia, hydromyelia

Gamut S-40

VERTEBRAL PEDICLE EROSION OR DESTRUCTION

COMMON
1. Intraspinal neoplasm or cyst (esp. neurofibroma, meningioma)
2. Metastasis
3. Tuberculosis, fungus$_g$, or other infectious disease

UNCOMMON
1. Benign bone tumor (eg, aneurysmal bone cyst, giant cell tumor, hemangiopericytoma)
2. [Congenital absence]
3. Eosinophilic granuloma (histiocytosis X$_g$)
4. Hydatid disease
5. Lymphoma$_g$
6. Multiple myeloma
7. Syringomyelia
8. Vertebral artery aneurysm or tortuosity (cervical spine); AV malformation

Gamut S-41

VERTEBRAL PEDICLE SCLEROSIS

COMMON
1. Metastasis (osteoblastic)
2. Osteoblastoma
3. Osteoid osteoma
4. Stress-induced
   a. Congenital absence or hypoplasia of contralateral posterior elements
   b. Malalignment of apophyseal joints
   c. Spondylolisthesis

UNCOMMON
1. Idiopathic
2. Lymphoma_g
3. Osteosarcoma; Ewing's sarcoma
4. Paget's disease
5. Posttraumatic (healed fracture)

References:
1. Pettine K, Klassen R: Osteoid osteoma and osteoblastoma of the spine. J Bone Joint Surg 1986;68A:354-361
2. Swischuk LE: Differential Diagnosis in Pediatric Radiology. Baltimore: Williams & Wilkins, 1984, p 396
3. Wilkinson RH, Hall JE: The sclerotic pedicle: Tumor or pseudotumor? Radiology 1974;111:683-688

Gamut S-42

SMALL OR NARROW INTERVERTEBRAL FORAMEN

COMMON
1. Degenerative or posttraumatic arthritis with hypertrophic bony ridging and spurring

UNCOMMON
1. Diastematomyelia
2. Fused vertebra
3. Klippel-Feil S.
4. Meningomyelocele
5. Posterior subluxation of cervical spine
6. Unilateral bar with scoliosis

Reference:
1. Swischuk LE: Differential Diagnosis in Pediatric Radiology. Baltimore: Williams & Wilkins, 1984, pp 418-419

Gamut S-43

ENLARGED INTERVERTEBRAL FORAMEN

COMMON

1. Neurofibroma

UNCOMMON

1. Congenital absence or hypoplasia of pedicle or neural arch
2. Dermoid, teratoma
3. Dejerine-Sottas S. (hypertrophic interstitial neuropathy)
4. Dural ectasia (eg, idiopathic, Marfan S., Ehlers- Danlos S.)
5. Fibroma of spinal ligaments
6. Hydatid disease
7. Lipoma
8. Lymphoma$_g$
9. Meningioma
10. Metastasis to spine or nerve
11. Neuroblastoma, ganglioneuroma
12. Neurofibromatosis (bony dysplasia, dural ectasia, lateral thoracic meningocele)
13. Posttraumatic (eg, fracture; traumatic avulsion of nerve root with "diverticulum"); postsurgical
14. Primary neoplasm of spine or spinal cord (eg, chordoma)
15. Spondylolysis
16. Vertebral artery aneurysm or tortuosity (eg, coarctation of aorta)

References:

1. Anderson RE, Shealy CN: Cervical pedicle erosion and rootlet compression caused by a tortuous vertebral artery. Radiology 1970;96:537-538
2. Danziger J, Bloch S: The widened cervical intervertebral foramen. Radiology 1975;116:671-674
3. Patel DV, Ferguson RJL, Schey WL: Enlargement of the intervertebral foramen, an unusual cause. AJR 1978;131: 911-913
4. Swischuk LE: Differential Diagnosis in Pediatric Radiology. Baltimore: Williams & Wilkins, 1984, pp 418-419

Gamut S-44

DEFECTIVE OR DESTROYED POSTERIOR NEURAL ARCHES

Congenital Defects

1. Defect in posterior arch of C1 (rarely C2 or other vertebrae)
2. Diastematomyelia
3. Meningocele, meningomyelocele, sacral dimple
4. [Normal synchondroses between body and arches]
5. Spina bifida occulta (usually L5 or S1) (See S-44A)

Acquired Defects or Destruction

1. Fracture with hyperextension injury (eg, hangman's fracture of C2)
2. Histiocytosis X_g
3. Hydatid disease
4. Metastasis
5. Multiple myeloma
6. Osteomyelitis
7. Primary neoplasm of spine (eg, hemangioma, aneurysmal bone cyst, osteoblastoma, sarcoma)
8. Spondylolysis, spondylolisthesis (pars interarticularis defects or fatigue fractures)

Reference:
1. Swischuk LE: Differential Diagnosis in Pediatric Radiology. Baltimore: Williams & Wilkins, 1984, pp 396-398

Subgamut S-44A

SPINA BIFIDA OCCULTA OR APERTA

Spina Bifida Occulta*

COMMON
1. Isolated anomaly

UNCOMMON
1. Dermoid; epidermoid cyst
2. Diastematomyelia
3. Filum terminale lipoma
4. Lipomeningocele
5. Tethered cord S.

* Skin-covered defect in posterior neural arch, commonly seen in the lower lumbar spine or upper sacrum and rarely associated with neurologic defect by itself.

Spina Bifida Aperta*

1. Meningocele
2. Meningomyelocele
3. Myeloschisis
4. Myelocystocele

* Incomplete fusion of posterior elements of vertebrae and overlying soft tissues, almost always associated with neurologic defect.

Reference:
1. Dahner W: Radiology Review Manual. Baltimore: Williams & Wilkins, 1991, p 95

SACRAL AGENESIS OR DEFORMITY

Agenesis or Hypoplasia

1. Caudal regression S. or mermaid S. (usually in infants of diabetic mothers)
2. Teratoma, presacral

Deformity (Curved or Sickle-Shaped Sacrum)

1. Imperforate anus
2. Meningocele (anterior, lateral, or intrasacral)
3. Teratoma, presacral
4. Tethered cord (often with spinal lipoma)

Reference:
1. Swischuk LE: Differential Diagnosis in Pediatric Radiology. Baltimore: Williams & Wilkins, 1984, pp 435-436

SACROILIAC JOINT DISEASE (EROSION, WIDENING, SCLEROSIS AND/OR FUSION)

COMMON
+*1. Ankylosing spondylitis
 *2. Infectious arthritis or osteomyelitis (eg, pyogenic, tuberculous)
+3. [Osteitis condensans ilii]
 4. Osteoarthritis, degenerative or posttraumatic
 5. Rheumatoid arthritis (incl. juvenile)

UNCOMMON

+1. Agenesis (caudal dysplasia)
  2. Bone neoplasm, primary (eg, chordoma, sarcoma) or metastatic
  3. Enteropathic arthritis due to inflammatory bowel disease (eg, ulcerative colitis, Crohn's disease, Whipple's disease)
  4. Familial Mediterranean fever
 *5. Gaucher's disease
  6. Gout
+7. Hyperparathyroidism, primary or secondary (renal osteodystrophy)
+8. Leukemia
+9. Multicentric reticulohistiocytosis (lipoid dermatoarthritis)
*10. Occupational acro-osteolysis (eg, polyvinylchloride osteolysis)
*11. Paraplegia, paralysis
 12. Pseudogout (CPPD crystal deposition disease)
 13. Pseudohypoparathyroidism
*14. Psoriatic arthritis
*15. Reiter S.
*16. Relapsing polychondritis
 17. Sacroiliitis circumscripta

+Bilateral symmetrical.
*Fusion of sacroiliac joint(s) may occur.

References:

1. Burgener FA, Kormano M: Differential Diagnosis in Conventional Radiology. (ed 2) New York: Thieme Medical Publ, 1991, p183
2. Resnik CS, Resnick D: Radiology of disorders of the sacroiliac joints. JAMA 1985;253:2863-2866

Gamut S-47

SACROCOCCYGEAL OR PRESACRAL MASS (See Gamut S-48)

COMMON

1. Abscess (eg, rectal perforation from trauma or surgery; sinus tract from Crohn's disease, ulcerative colitis, amebiasis, schistosomiasis, tuberculosis, or lymphogranuloma venereum)
2. Bone cyst or neoplasm, benign (eg, aneurysmal bone cyst, giant cell tumor)
3. Carcinoma of prostate
4. Hematoma; fracture
5. Malignant neoplasm of sacrum (eg, chordoma, sarcoma, metastasis, myeloma)
6. [Normal variant; pelvic surgery]
7. Teratoma; dermoid cyst

UNCOMMON

1. Arachnoid, extradural, or perineural cyst
2. [Ectopic kidney]
3. Hamartoma
4. Hydatid cyst
5. Hydroureter; urinoma
6. Intraspinal neoplasm, other (eg, ependymoma, lipoma)
7. Lymphocele
8. Lymphoma$_g$
9. Meningocele, anterior sacral
10. Neurenteric cyst
11. Neurogenic tumor
12. Osteomyelitis of sacrum
13. Ovarian cyst or neoplasm; tubovarian abscess
14. Rectal duplication
15. Spindle cell tumor$_g$

References:
1. Epstein BS: The Spine. (ed 4) Philadelphia: Lea & Febiger, 1976
2. Lombardi G, Passerini A: Spinal Cord Diseases: A Radiologic and Myelographic Analysis. Baltimore: Williams & Wilkins, 1964

3. Silverman FN (ed): Caffey's Pediatric X-ray Diagnosis. (ed 8) Chicago: Year Book Medical Publ, 1985
4. Werner JL, Taybi H: Presacral masses in childhood. AJR 1970;109:403-410

Gamut S-48

PRIMARY NEOPLASM OF THE SACRUM
Benign

COMMON
1. Giant cell tumor

UNCOMMON
1. Aneurysmal bone cyst
2. Osteoblastoma
3. Osteochondroma
4. Osteoma

Malignant

COMMON
1. Chordoma

UNCOMMON
1. Chondrosarcoma
2. Ewing's sarcoma
3. Fibrosarcoma; malignant fibrous histiocytoma
4. Lymphoma$_g$
5. Malignant giant cell tumor
6. Neurogenic sarcoma
7. Osteosarcoma
8. Paget's sarcoma
9. Plasmacytoma
10. Radiation-induced sarcoma
11. Spindle cell neoplasm$_g$

Reference:
1. Smith J: International Skeletal Society Lecture. Philadelphia, 1984

NARROW DISK SPACES

COMMON
1. Ankylosing spondylitis
2. Block vertebra, congenital or acquired (See S-25)
*3. Degenerative disk disease (usually associated with osteoarthritis)
*4. Herniated disk
5. Kyphosis, scoliosis (severe)
*6. Neuropathic arthropathy (eg, diabetes, syringomyelia, tabes dorsalis)
*7. Osteomyelitis (eg, pyogenic, tuberculous, sarcoid, brucellar, typhoid)
*8. Rheumatoid arthritis; other inflammatory arthritis
9. Scheuermann's disease

UNCOMMON
1. Cockayne S.
2. Discitis, spondyloarthritis (childhood)
3. Kniest dysplasia
4. Morquio S.
5. Neoplasm (rarely)
*6. Ochronosis (alkaptonuria)
*7. Pseudogout (CPPD crystal deposition disease)
8. Spondyloepiphyseal dysplasia
*9. Trauma (flexion-rotation injury)

*Often with adjacent sclerosis of the vertebral margins.

Reference:
1. Swischuk LE: Differential Diagnosis in Pediatric Radiology. Baltimore: Williams & Wilkins, 1984, pp 424-426

Gamut S-50

WIDE DISK SPACES

1. Acromegaly
2. Biconcave vertebrae, other causes (See S-19)
3. Gaucher's disease
4. Osteomalacia
5. Osteoporosis
6. Platyspondyly (esp. Morquio S., osteogenesis imperfecta, cretinism) (See S-15)
7. Sickle cell anemia
8. Trauma (hyperextension injury to spine)

Gamut S-51

CALCIFICATION OF ONE OR MORE INTERVERTEBRAL DISKS

COMMON
1. Degenerative spondylosis
2. Idiopathic (eg, transient calcification in children; persistent type in adults)
3. Ochronosis (alkaptonuria)
4. Posttraumatic
5. Spinal fusion (eg, congenital block vertebra, Klippel-Feil S., myositis ossificans progressiva, surgical fusion)

UNCOMMON
1. Aarskog S.
2. Ankylosing spondylitis
3. Cockayne S.
4. Diffuse idiopathic skeletal hyperostosis (DISH)
5. Gout
6. Hemochromatosis
7. Homocystinuria

8. Hypercalcemia
9. Hyperparathyroidism
10. Hypervitaminosis D
11. Hypophosphatasia
12. Infection (eg, brucellosis)
13. Paraplegia; poliomyelitis
14. Pseudogout (CPPD crystal deposition disease)
15. Rheumatoid spondylitis (incl. juvenile chronic arthritis)
16. Spondyloepiphyseal dysplasia tarda

References:

1. Dussault RG, Kaye JJ: Intervertebral disk calcification associated with spine fusion. Radiology 1977;125:57-61
2. Edeiken J, Dalinka M, Karasick D: Edeiken's Roentgen Diagnosis of Diseases of Bone. (ed 4) Baltimore: Williams & Wilkins, 1989
3. Greenfield GB: Radiology of Bone Diseases. (ed 5) Philadelphia: Lippincott, 1990
4. Kozlowski K, Beighton P: Gamut Index of Skeletal Dysplasias. Berlin: Springer-Verlag, 1984, pp 48-49
5. Mainzer F: Herniation of the nucleus pulposus. A rare complication of intervertebral-disk calcification in children. Radiology 1973;107:167-170
6. Murray RO, Jacobson HG, Stoker D: The Radiology of Skeletal Disorders. (ed 3) Edinburgh: Churchill Livingstone, 1990
7. Swischuk LE: Differential Diagnosis in Pediatric Radiology. Baltimore: Williams & Wilkins, 1984, p 427
8. Taybi H, Lachman RS: Radiology of Syndromes, Metabolic Disorders, and Skeletal Dysplasias. (ed 3) Chicago: Year Book Medical Publ, 1990, p 880
9. Weinberger A, Myers AR: Intervertebral disc calcification in adults: a review. Semin Arthritis Rheum 1978;18:69-75

Gamut S-52

GAS IN AN INTERVERTEBRAL DISK (VACUUM DISK)

COMMON

1. Degenerative disk disease; spondylosis deformans

UNCOMMON
1. Fractured vertebra
2. Osteomyelitis of vertebra (rare)
3. Osteonecrosis with vertebral collapse (Kümmell's disease)
4. Schmorl's nodes (on CT)

Reference:
1. Greenfield GB: Radiology of Bone Diseases. (ed 5) Philadelphia: Lippincott, 1990

Gamut S-53

SYNDROMES WITH A NARROW SPINAL CANAL (NARROW INTERPEDICULAR DISTANCE): SPINAL STENOSIS

COMMON
1. Achondroplasia, hypochondroplasia
2. Acromegaly
3. Diastrophic dysplasia
4. Klippel-Feil S.

UNCOMMON
1. Acrodysostosis
2. Acromesomelic dysplasia
3. Arteriohepatic S. (Alagille S.)
4. Cauda equina S. (narrow lumbar spinal canal S.)
5. Dyschondrosteosis
6. Gordon S.
7. Kniest dysplasia
8. Osteoglophonic dwarfism
9. Pseudogout
10. Pseudohypoparathyroidism, pseudopseudohypoparathyroidism
11. Smith-McCort S.

12. Thanatophoric dysplasia
13. Weill-Marchesani S.

References:
1. Kozlowski K, Beighton P: Gamut Index of Skeletal Dysplasias. Berlin: Springer-Verlag, 1984, pp 47-48
2. Taybi H, Lachman RS: Radiology of Syndromes, Metabolic Disorders, and Skeletal Dysplasias. (ed 3) Chicago: Year Book Medical Publ, 1990, p 880

WIDE SPINAL CANAL (INCREASED INTERPEDICULAR DISTANCE) (See Gamuts S-55 and S-57)

COMMON
1. Intraspinal neoplasm (eg, ependymoma, astrocytoma, neurofibroma, lipoma) or cyst
2. Meningocele, meningomyelocele
3. [Rotation of vertebra due to scoliosis or poor radiographic positioning]

UNCOMMON
1. AV malformation
2. Diastematomyelia
3. Idiopathic
4. Marfan S.
5. Mucopolysaccharidoses (esp. Hurler S., Hunter S., Morquio S.)
6. Neurofibromatosis, dural ectasia
7. Otopalatodigital S.
8. Syringomyelia, hydromyelia
9. Tethered cord S.

Gamut S-55

INTRAMEDULLARY LESION (WIDENING OF SPINAL CORD ON MYELOGRAPHY, CT, OR MRI) (See Gamuts M-99 to M-103)

COMMON

1. [Extrinsic compression (eg, by cervical ridge, herniated disk, large extramedullary or extradural tumor)]
2. Inflammation (eg, abscess; myelitis—viral or bacterial; multiple sclerosis)
3. Intramedullary tumor (esp. ependymoma and astrocytoma; also ganglioglioma, hemangioblastoma, primary melanoma)
4. Syringomyelia, hydromyelia (see S-55A)

UNCOMMON

1. AV malformation, angioma
2. Dermoid; teratoma; epidermoid
3. Diastematomyelia
4. Granuloma (eg, sarcoidosis, tuberculosis)
5. Hematoma, contusion, or edema of cord; anticoagulant therapy
6. Lipoma
7. Lymphoma$_g$
8. Metastasis (eg, breast, lung, melanoma); drop metastasis through the central canal (eg, medulloblastoma)
9. Myelomeningocele
10. [Postradiation myelopathy]
11. [Spinal cord atrophy (See S-56)]

References:

1. Epstein BS: Spinal canal mass lesions. Radiol Clin North Am 1966;4:185-202
2. Epstein BS: The Spine: A Radiological Text and Atlas. (ed 4) Philadelphia: Lea & Febiger, 1976
3. Lewtas N: The Spine and Myelography. In: Sutton D (ed), Textbook of Radiology and Imaging. (ed 4) Edinburgh: Churchill Livingstone, 1987

4. Moseley IF: Myelography. In: du Boulay GH (ed), A Text-book of Radiological Diagnosis. (ed 5) London: HK Lewis, 1984

5. Stevens JM: The Spine and Spinal Cord. In: Sutton D, Young JWR (eds): A Short Textbook of Clinical Imaging. London: Springer-Verlag, 1990, pp 806-811

Subgamut S-55A

CAUSES OF SYRINGOMYELIA OR HYDROMYELIA

1. Arachnoiditis
2. Chiari I, Chiari II (Arnold Chiari) malformation
3. Herniation of cerebellar tonsils through foramen magnum due to posterior fossa mass
4. Posttraumatic
5. Spinal stenosis
6. Tumor (rostral or caudal to cyst; intra- or extramedullary)

Reference:

1. Houghton V, et al: Chapter 40, In: Stark DD, Bradley WG (eds): Magnetic Resonance Imaging. (ed 2) St. Louis: CV Mosby, 1992

Gamut S-56

SPINAL CORD ATROPHY

COMMON
1. Multiple sclerosis
2. Posttraumatic
3. Spondylosis; disk hernation (esp. cervical)
4. Syringomyelia, hydromyelia (after collapse)

UNCOMMON

1. Amyotrophic lateral sclerosis
2. AV malformation of cord
3. Friedreich's ataxia
4. Ischemia with cord infarction
5. Other motor neuron disease or motor and sensory neuropathies
6. Postradiation therapy myelopathy
7. Subacute combined degeneration
8. Tabes dorsalis

Reference:

1. Stevens JM: The Spine and Spinal Cord. In: Sutton D, Young JWR (eds): A Short Textbook of Clinical Imaging. London: Springer-Verlag, 1990, p 811

Gamut S-57

SMALL SPINAL CORD

FOCALLY SMALL CORD

1. Bony spinal stenosis
2. Collapsed syrinx
3. Compression due to herniated disk, epidural tumor, or extramedullary mass (eg, arachnoid cyst)
4. Multiple sclerosis
5. Myelomalacia
6. Postinfarction of cord
7. Postradiation therapy myelopathy
8. Postsurgical
9. Posttraumatic

DIFFUSELY SMALL CORD

1. Atrophy
2. Collapsed syrinx
3. Cord tethering
4. Cord transection

5. Kyphoscoliosis
6. Multiple sclerosis (diffuse)
7. Postoperative (caudal to level of previous surgery)
8. Postradiation therapy myelopathy

References:

1. Houghton V, et al: Chapter 40, In: Stark DD, Bradley WG (eds): Magnetic Resonance Imaging. (ed 2) St. Louis: CV Mosby, 1992
2. Shoukimas GM: Chapter 41, In: Stark DD, Bradley WG (eds): Magnetic Resonance Imaging. (ed 2) St. Louis: CV Mosby, 1992

Gamut S-58

INTRADURAL, EXTRAMEDULLARY LESION (ON MYELOGRAPHY, CT, OR MRI) (See Gamuts M-104 to M-108)

COMMON

1. Arachnoiditis (see S-58A)
2. Meningioma
3. Metastasis, esp. leptomeningeal seeding from CNS tumor (eg, medulloblastoma, glioblastoma, pinealoma, ependymoma) or hematogenous from lung, breast, melanoma, lymphoma$_g$
4. Neurofibroma

UNCOMMON

1. Arachnoid cyst
2. Cysticercosis (cysts)
3. Dermoid, teratoma; neuroectodermal cyst; epidermoid cyst
4. Ependymoma of conus medullaris
5. Granuloma (eg, tuberculoma; fungal—aspergilloma; sarcoid)

6. Hemangioblastoma; hemangiopericytoma
7. Lipoma (lipomyeloschisis)
8. Meningocele
9. [Tortuosity of nerve roots]
10. Vascular malformation; angioma; varices

Reference:
1. Stevens JM: The Spine and Spinal Cord. In: Sutton D, Young JWR (eds): A Short Textbook of Clinical Imaging. London: Springer-Verlag, 1990, pp 802-806

Subgamut S-58A

ARACHNOIDITIS

1. Cysticercosis
2. Pantopaque myelography
3. Postoperative
4. Posttraumatic
5. Spinal meningitis (eg, bacterial, tuberculous, fungal, sarcoid, HIV 1 infection)

Gamut S-59

EXTRADURAL LESION (ON MYELOGRAPHY, CT, OR MRI) (See Gamuts M-109, M-110)

COMMON
1. Dermoid, teratoma, epidermoid
2. Epidural metastasis (eg, lymphoma$_g$)
3. Epidural scar (eg, after disk surgery)
4. Fracture fragment or dislocation from vertebral trauma

5. Hematoma, traumatic or spontaneous
6. Herniated disk
7. [Iatrogenic (needle point defect, extradural injection of Pantopaque)]
8. Ligamentum flavum thickening; intraspinal ligament - ossification (eg, DISH; primary—esp. in Japanese)
9. Lipomatosis (obesity, steroid therapy, Cushing S.)
10. Meningioma (with intradural component)
11. Metastasis (esp. carcinoma of lung, breast, prostate, colon)
12. Neurogenic tumor (eg, neurofibroma)
13. Osteomyelitis, epidural abscess (esp. tuberculous, pyogenic)
14. Spinal stenosis; spondylosis; osteophyte
15. Vertebral neoplasm with intraspinal extension (eg, sarcoma, myeloma, chordoma, hemangioma, giant cell tumor, aneurysmal bone cyst, osteoblastoma, osteochondroma)

UNCOMMON

1. Amyloidosis
2. Arachnoid cyst
3. Arachnoiditis (See S-58A)
4. Epidural granuloma (eg, tuberculous, fungal$_g$, sarcoid)
5. Extramedullary hematopoiesis
6. Lipoma
7. Osteoporosis with fracture and granulation tissue
8. Paget's disease (uncalcified osteoid)
9. Parasitic infection (eg, cysticercosis, hydatid disease, schistosomiasis)
10. Retroperitoneal neoplasm extending through inter-vertebral foramen (eg, neuroblastoma, lymphoma$_g$)

References:
1. Du Boulay GH (ed): A Textbook of X-Ray Diagnosis by British Authors. Neuroradiology. London: AK Lewis, 1984
2. Epstein BS: Spinal canal mass lesions. Radiol Clin North Am 1966;4:185-202
3. Houghton V, et al: Chapter 40, In: Stark DD, Bradley WG (eds): Magnetic Resonance Imaging. (ed 2) St. Louis: CV Mosby, 1992

4. Shoukimas GM: Chapter 41, In: Stark DD, Bradley WG (eds): Magnetic Resonance Imaging. (ed 2) St. Louis: CV Mosby, 1992

5. Stevens JM: The Spine and Spinal Cord. In: Sutton D, Young JWR (eds): A Short Textbook of Clinical Imaging. London: Springer-Verlag, 1990, pp 791-802

6. Taveras JM, Wood EH: Diagnostic Neuroradiology. (ed 2) Baltimore: Williams & Wilkins, 1976

Gamut S-60

SPINAL BLOCK (ON MYELOGRAPHY, CT, OR MRI)

COMMON

1. Fracture, traumatic or pathologic
2. Hemorrhage (traumatic, spontaneous, anticoagulant therapy)
3. Herniated disk
4. Metastasis or contiguous spread of malignancy
5. Neoplasm of spine, primary (eg, sarcoma, myeloma, chordoma, giant cell tumor)
6. Neurogenic tumor (esp. neurofibroma)
7. Spinal stenosis

UNCOMMON

1. Abscess, epidural
2. Achondroplasia
3. Arachnoiditis (See S-58A)
4. Cyst of spinal canal (eg, congenital, arachnoid, dermoid, cysticercus, hydatid)
5. Fibrous dysplasia
6. Granuloma (eg, tuberculosis, schistosomiasis)
7. Hemangioma of vertebra
8. Intramedullary lesion, large (eg, syringomyelia, ependymoma, lipoma)
9. Klippel-Feil S.

10. Lipoma of canal
11. Lymphoma$_g$
12. Meningioma
13. Osteomyelitis of spine
14. Paget's disease

References:
1. Greenfield GB: Radiology of Bone Diseases. (ed 5) Philadelphia: Lippincott, 1990
2. O'Carroll MP, Witcombe JB: Primary disorders of bone with "spinal block." Clin Radiol 1979;30:299-306

Gamut S-61

TORTUOUS FILLING DEFECT ON LUMBAR MYELOGRAPHY

COMMON
1. Nerve root elongation, redundancy, or displacement (eg, spinal stenosis or arthrosis, disk herniation, achondroplasia)

UNCOMMON
1. Arachnoiditis (See S-58A)
2. Extradural or intradural neoplasm
3. Multiple lesions at same or adjacent levels
4. Vascular abnormality (eg, AV malformation, venous angioma, varices)

Reference:
1. Cronquist S, Thulin C-A: Significance of tortuous filling defects at lumbar myelography. Acta Radiologica Diag 1979; 20:561-568

MRI Based Gamuts

M

MRI (Magnetic Resonance Imaging) Introduction

The organization of the MR gamuts is heavily based on the appearance of lesions on T1- and T2-weighted images. For those readers less familiar with magnetic resonance imaging, let me add that a T1-weighted spin echo image is one with a short repetition time (TR) and a short echo delay time (TE) (which are both operator-selectable imaging parameters). ("Short" in the context of TR is less than 500 msec and "short" in the context of TE is ideally less than 20 msec — for a high-field system — or 30 msec for a low or mid field system.) T1-weighted gradient echo images are acquired with flip angles larger than $45°$ and echo delay times generally less than 10 msec. If the repetition times are less than 200 msec, then either RF or gradient spoiling should be used. Such T1-weighted gradient echo techniques are known as FLASH (Siemens), SPGR (for spoiled GRASS, GE), or RF-Spoiled FAST (Picker).

T2-weighted spin echo images are those produced with a long TR and a long TE. "Long" in the context of TR is greater than 2,000 msec for applications outside the brain at any field strength. For brain imaging, a long TR at 0.5 Tesla (or below) is 2,000 msec while above 0.5 Tesla the TR should be in the 2,500-3,000 msec range for a T2-weighted image. "Long" in the context of TE is generally on the order of 80 msec or greater. While gradient echo images are never truly T2-weighted, there are certain parameter adjustments that can increase the T2 (or, more correctly, T2*) influence on image contrast. These include a long TE (greater than 18 msec), a short TR (less than 100 msec *without* spoiling), and a low flip angle (less than 30°). (While the low flip angle actually results in proton density weighting, T2 and proton density tend to track together in disease.)

The organization of the MR gamuts is slightly different than that of the preceding, x-ray-based Gamuts. The reader is therefore advised to become familiar with the main, organ system-based organization as well as the suborganization for the brain prior to extensive use.

Finally, I wish to acknowledge the authors of many of the clinical chapters in the textbook *Magnetic Resonance Imaging* (2nd edition) edited by David Stark and myself (Mosby-Year Book Co., St. Louis, MO,1992) who inadvertently contributed to the gamuts that follow. I also owe a great deal of thanks to my personal assistant of nine years, Kaye Finley, for the untold hours spent in formatting, reformatting, editing, and reorganizing this material. Without her help over many evenings and weekends, this project would not have been possible.

William G. Bradley, Jr., M.D., Ph.D., F.A.C.R.

M

MRI

BRAIN

PARENCHYMAL

Dark on T1-weighted image, bright on T2-weighted image

Nonspecific location
   No mass effect
      Nonenhancing (M-1)
      Enhancing (M-2)
   Mass effect
      Nonenhancing (M-3)
         Causes of dural sinus thrombosis (M-3A)
         Causes of vasculitis (M-3B)
      Enhancing (M-4)
Subependymal
   Nonenhancing (M-5)
   Enhancing (M-6)
      Subependymal tumor spread (M-6A)
Periventricular
   No mass effect
      Nonenhancing (M-7)
      Enhancing (M-8)
         Periventricular disease in AIDS (M-8A)
         Leukodystrophies (M-8B)
   Mass effect
      Nonenhancing (M-9)
      Enhancing (M-10)

M

Cortical
No mass effect
Nonenhancing (M-33)
Enhancing (M-34)
Mass effect (M-35)
Basal ganglia (M-36)
Intravascular (M-37)
Brain stem (M-38)

Bright on T1-weighted image and T2-weighted image
Nonspecific location (M-39)
Sella region (M-40)

Bright on T1-weighted image, dark on T2-weighted image
Nonspecific location (M-41)
Sella region (M-42)

Signal void
Nonspecific location (M-43)
Subependymal (M-44)
Brain stem (M-45)
Sella region (M-46)

M

VENTRICLES AND INTRAVENTRICULAR LESIONS

Ventricles
Small ventricles, small sulci (M-47)
Enlarged ventricles, small sulci (M-48)
Causes of communicating hydrocephalus (M-48A)
(See also B-48)
Causes of obstructive hydrocephalus (M-48B)
(See also B-48)
Enlarged ventricles, enlarged sulci (M-49)
Abnormal ventricular configuration (M-50)

Intraventricular mass
CSF intensity (M-51)
Dark on T1-weighted image, bright on T2-weighted image
Nonenhancing (M-52)
Enhancing (M-53)

Dark on T1-weighted image and T2-weighted image (M-54)

Bright on T1-weighted image (M-55)

Intraventricular signal void (M-56)

EXTRAAXIAL LESIONS

Subarachnoid space
Isointense to brain (M-57)
Hyperintense to brain (M-58)
Isointense to CSF (M-59)
Signal void (M-60)
Mass in the cerebellopontine angle cistern (M-61)

Leptomeningeal
Focal enhancement (M-62)
Diffuse enhancement (M-63)

Pachymeningeal (dural)
Nonenhancing lesion (M-64)
Enhancing lesion (M-65)

Extraaxial fluid collection
CSF intensity (M-66)
Dark on T1-weighted image (M-67)
Bright on T1-weighted image (M-68)

Extraaxial mass
Nonenhancing (M-69)
Enhancing (M-70)

Extracranial mass
CSF intensity (M-71)
Dark on T1-weighted image (M-72)
Bright on T1-weighted image (M-73)

ORBIT

Lesion of the globe (M-74)

Lesion of the optic nerve/nerve sheath (M-75)

Retrobulbar mass (M-76)

Extraocular muscle enlargement (M-77)

Lateral extraconal lesion (M-78)

Enlarged superior ophthalmic vein (M-79)

Thrombosis of superior ophthalmic vein (M-80)

Orbital wall lesion (M-81)

PARANASAL SINUSES

Sinonasal mass without bone changes
    Bright on T2-weighted image (M-82)
    Dark on T2-weighted image (M-83)

Sinonasal mass with bony remodeling without erosion (M-84)

Sinonasal mass with bony erosion (M-85)

Vascular sinonasal mass with flow voids (M-86)

Fibro-osseous lesion of a paranasal sinus (M-87)

M

HEAD AND NECK

Skull base lesion (M-88)

Nasopharyngeal mass (M-89)

Parapharyngeal mass
    Prestyloid (M-90)
    Poststyloid (M-91)

Tongue/oral cavity mass (M-92)

Salivary gland lesion (M-93)
    Causes of intraparotid lymphadenopathy (M-93A)

Mass of the hypopharynx or larynx (M-94)

Neck mass (M-95)

SPINE

VERTEBRAL BODY ABNORMALITIES

Focal
Decreased signal on T1-weighted image and increased signal on T2-weighted image (M-96)
High signal on T1-weighted image (M-97)

Diffuse (M-98)

INTRAMEDULLARY LESION (See also Gamut S-55)

CSF intensity (M-99)

Dark on T1-weighted images, bright on T2-weighted image
No mass effect (M-100)
Mass effect (M-101)

Dark on T1 and T2-weighted images
Mass effect (M-102)

Bright on T1-weighted image (M-103)

EXTRAMEDULLARY, INTRADURAL LESION (See also Gamut S-58)

CSF intensity (M-104)

Dark on T1-weighted image, bright on T2-weighted image
No mass effect (M-105)
Mass effect (M-106)
Sources of drop metastases to spinal subarachnoid space (M-106A)

Bright on T1-weighted image, dark on T2-weighted image (M-107)

Signal void (M-108)

EXTRADURAL LESION (See also Gamut S-59)

With normal adjacent bone (M-109)

With abnormal adjacent bone (M-110)

Gamut M-1

PARENCHYMAL DISEASE

DARK ON T1-WEIGHTED IMAGE, BRIGHT ON T2-WEIGHTED IMAGE, NONSPECIFIC LOCATION, NO MASS EFFECT, NONENHANCING

1. Carbon monoxide poisoning
2. Gliosis (following trauma, infarct, infection)
3. Low-grade glioma
4. Multiple sclerosis
5. Shearing injury
6. Tuberous sclerosis (high parietal)

Gamut M-2

PARENCHYMAL DISEASE

DARK ON T1-WEIGHTED IMAGE, BRIGHT ON T2-WEIGHTED IMAGE, NONSPECIFIC LOCATION, NO MASS EFFECT, ENHANCING

1. [Flow artifact]
2. Indolent infection
3. Multiple sclerosis
4. [Normal vein]
5. Small glioma
6. Small metastasis
7. Small vascular malformation

Gamut M-3

PARENCHYMAL DISEASE

DARK ON T1-WEIGHTED IMAGE, BRIGHT ON T2-WEIGHTED IMAGE, NONSPECIFIC LOCATION, MASS EFFECT, NONENHANCING

1. Acute stroke
2. Contusion
3. Cryptococcoma (toruloma)
4. Hyperacute hemorrhage
5. Low-grade glioma
6. Viral encephalitis

Subgamut M-3A

CAUSES OF DURAL SINUS THROMBOSIS

1. Antithrombin III deficiency
2. Birth control pills
3. Congestive heart failure
4. Dehydration
5. Disseminated intravascular coagulation (DIC)
6. Infection
7. Lupus anticoagulant
8. Malignant invasion
9. Polycythemia vera
10. Pregnancy
11. Primary vasculitis
12. Sickle cell disease
13. Thrombocytosis
14. Vascular malformation

Reference:
1. Brant-Zawadzki M, Chapter 21, In: Stark DD, Bradley WG (eds): Magnetic Resonance Imaging. (ed 2) St. Louis: CV Mosby, 1992

Subgamut M-3B

CAUSES OF VASCULITIS

1. Amphetamine/cocaine abuse
2. Behcet's disease
3. Collagen vascular disease (eg, lupus)
4. Giant cell arteritis (common)
5. Granulomatosis angiitis (rare)
6. Infection (eg, herpes, TB, syphilis [rare])
7. Migraine
8. Polyarteritis nodosum
9. Radiation therapy
10. Sarcoidosis
11. Takayasu's arteritis

Reference:
1. Brant-Zawadzki M, Chapter 21, In: Stark DD, Bradley WG (eds): Magnetic Resonance Imaging. (ed 2) St. Louis: CV Mosby, 1992

Gamut M-4

DARK ON T1-WEIGHTED IMAGE, BRIGHT ON T2-WEIGHTED IMAGE, NONSPECIFIC LOCATION, MASS EFFECT, ENHANCING

1. Abscess
2. Cerebritis
3. Ganglion cell tumors (rare)
4. High-grade glioma
5. Metastasis
6. Lymphoma (primary or metastatic)
7. PNET (primitive neuroectodermal tumor)
8. Radiation necrosis
9. Tumefactive multiple sclerosis

Gamut M-5

DARK ON T1-WEIGHTED IMAGE, BRIGHT ON T2-WEIGHTED IMAGE, SUBEPENDYMAL, NONENHANCING

SMOOTH
1. Centrally tracking vasogenic edema
2. Interstitial edema (transependymal resorption of CSF)
3. Ischemic gliosis/demyelination
4. [Normal caudate body]
5. Subependymal demyelination after interstitial edema

LUMPY
1. Hamartomas of tuberous sclerosis
2. Heterotopic gray matter

Gamut M-6

DARK ON T1-WEIGHTED IMAGE, BRIGHT ON T2-WEIGHTED IMAGE, SUBEPENDYMAL, ENHANCING

SMOOTH
1. Subependymal tumor spread (early) (See M-6A)
2. Ventriculitis/ependymitis

LUMPY
1. Giant cell astrocytoma (tuberous sclerosis)
2. Subependymal tumor spread (late) (See M-6A)

Subgamut M-6A

SUBEPENDYMAL TUMOR SPREAD

1. Ependymoma
2. Glioblastoma
3. Lymphoma
4. Medulloblastoma
5. Metastasis (esp. breast, lung, melanoma)

Gamut M-7

DARK ON T1-WEIGHTED IMAGE, BRIGHT ON T2-WEIGHTED IMAGE, PERIVENTRICULAR, NO MASS EFFECT, NONENHANCING

Patient Under 40

COMMON
1. HIV encephalitis (See M-8A)
2. Migraine
3. Multiple sclerosis
4. Systemic lupus erythematosus

UNCOMMON
1. Lyme disease
2. Periventricular leukomalacia
3. Postviral leukoencephalopathy (acute disseminated encephalomyelitis)

RARE
1. Leukodystrophies (See M-8B)
2. Marchiafava-Bignami disease
3. Subacute sclerosing panencephalitis (SSPE)

Patient Over 40

1. Deep white matter ischemia/infarction
2. Multiple sclerosis
3. [Normal (ependymitis granularis)]
4. Postirradiation

Nonspecific with Respect to Age

1. Diffuse necrotizing leukoencephalopathy (DNL)
2. Hamartomas of tuberous sclerosis
3. Heterotopic gray matter
4. Neurofibromatosis
5. [Normal late myelinating fibers (thalamoparietal tracts)]
6. Shearing injury

Gamut M-8

DARK ON T1-WEIGHTED IMAGE, BRIGHT ON T2-WEIGHTED IMAGE, PERIVENTRICULAR, NO MASS EFFECT, ENHANCING

1. Early metastatic disease
2. Early toxoplasmosis (See M-8A)
3. Leukodystrophies (enhancing active border [rare])
4. Subacute infarction

Subgamut M-8A

PERIVENTRICULAR DISEASE IN AIDS

1. Cytomegalic virus (CMV) infection
2. HIV encephalitis
3. Kaposi's sarcoma
4. Lymphoma$_g$
5. Progressive multifocal leukoencephalopathy (PML)
6. Toxoplasmosis

Subgamut M-8B

LEUKODYSTROPHIES

MACROCEPHALY (IN INFANT)
1. Alexander's disease (anterior, sparing of internal capsule, enhances with gadolinium)
2. Canavan's disease (peripheral to central, early involvement of subcortical U-fibers)

NORMOCEPHALY
1. Adrenoleukodystrophy (posterior, male, enhances with gadolinium)
2. Krabbe's disease (central to peripheral, nonenhancing)
3. Metachromatic leukodystrophy (central to peripheral, nonenhancing)
4. Pelizaeus-Merzbacher's disease (males, central to peripheral, nonenhancing, brain stem atrophy)

Reference:
1. Dietrich RB, In: Stark DD, Bradley WG (eds): Magnetic Resonance Imaging. (ed 2) St. Louis: CV Mosby, 1992

Gamut M-9

DARK ON T1-WEIGHTED IMAGE, BRIGHT ON T2-WEIGHTED IMAGE, PERIVENTRICULAR, MASS EFFECT, NONENHANCING

1. Hamartoma of tuberous sclerosis or neurofibromatosis
2. Infarction from vasculitis
3. Postviral leukoencephalopathy (ADEM)
4. Sickle cell infarcts
5. Visual pathway glioma (neurofibromatosis)

Gamut M-10

DARK ON T1-WEIGHTED IMAGE, BRIGHT ON T2-WEIGHTED IMAGE, PERIVENTRICULAR, MASS EFFECT, ENHANCING

1. Abscess (eg, CMV, toxoplasmosis)
2. Degenerated visual pathway glioma (neurofibromatosis)
3. Giant cell astrocytoma (tuberous sclerosis)
4. Intraventricular drop metastasis (eg, from glioblastoma)
5. Lymphoma$_g$
6. Metastatic disease
7. Tumefactive multiple sclerosis

Gamut M-11

DARK ON T1-WEIGHTED IMAGE, BRIGHT ON T2-WEIGHTED IMAGE, SUBCORTICAL, NO MASS EFFECT, NONENHANCING

1. Embolic infarction (See M-14A)
2. Progressive multifocal leukoencephalopathy (PML)
3. Shearing injury (nonhemorrhagic)

Gamut M-12

DARK ON T1-WEIGHTED IMAGE, BRIGHT ON T2-WEIGHTED IMAGE, SUBCORTICAL, NO MASS EFFECT, ENHANCING

1. Leptomeningeal carcinomatosis
2. Lymphoma$_g$
3. Meningitis (bacterial, occasionally fungal and viral)
4. Sarcoidosis

Gamut M-13

DARK ON T1-WEIGHTED IMAGE, BRIGHT ON T2-WEIGHTED IMAGE, SUBCORTICAL, MASS EFFECT, NONENHANCING

1. Heterotopic gray matter
2. Low-grade glioma
3. Progressive multifocal leukoencephalopathy (PML)

Gamut M-14

DARK ON T1-WEIGHTED IMAGE, BRIGHT ON T2-WEIGHTED IMAGE, SUBCORTICAL, MASS EFFECT, ENHANCING

1. Abscess
2. Emboli (See M-14A)
3. Metastases
4. Multiple sclerosis
5. Sarcoidosis

Subgamut M-14A

CAUSES OF CEREBRAL EMBOLI

SOURCE DISTAL TO LUNGS
1. Emboli (from cardiac mural thrombus, carotid dissection, open heart surgery, post angiogram)
2. Infection (infective endocarditis/subacute bacterial endocarditis [SBE])
3. Platelet emboli (from ulcerated carotid plaque)
4. Thrombi
5. Tumor (atrial myxoma, chorioepithelioma, marantic endocarditis)

SOURCE PROXIMAL TO LUNGS (REQUIRES RIGHT TO LEFT SHUNT [RARE])
1. Amniotic fluid embolism
2. Fat emboli (following trauma)
3. Thrombi (from inferior vena cava or other thrombophlebitis)

Gamut M-15

DARK ON T1-WEIGHTED IMAGE, BRIGHT ON T2-WEIGHTED IMAGE, CORTICAL, NO MASS EFFECT, NONENHANCING

1. Postinfarct
2. Postbleed
3. Postinfection
4. Postoperative defect/encephalomalacia
5. Posttrauma

Gamut M-16

DARK ON T1-WEIGHTED IMAGE, BRIGHT ON T2-WEIGHTED IMAGE, CORTICAL, NO MASS EFFECT, ENHANCING

1. Leptomeningeal carcinomatosis
2. Lymphoma$_g$
3. Meningitis
4. Subacute infarct

Gamut M-17

DARK ON T1-WEIGHTED IMAGE, BRIGHT ON T2-WEIGHTED IMAGE, CORTICAL, MASS EFFECT, NONENHANCING

1. Acute infarct
2. Low-grade glioma

Gamut M-18

DARK ON T1-WEIGHTED IMAGE, BRIGHT ON T2-WEIGHTED IMAGE, CORTICAL, MASS EFFECT, ENHANCING

1. Acute infarct (vascular enhancement secondary to slow flow)
2. Leptomeningeal metastases
3. Subacute infarct (gyral enhancement)

Gamut M-19

DARK ON T1-WEIGHTED IMAGE, BRIGHT ON T2-WEIGHTED IMAGE, BASAL GANGLIA

COMMON
1. Ischemia-anoxia (eg, near-drowning)
2. Lacunar infarcts
3. Multiple sclerosis

UNCOMMON
1. Carbon monoxide poisoning
2. Methanol intoxication
3. Behcet's disease
4. Leigh's disease (necrotizing encephalopathy)

Gamut M-20

DARK ON T1-WEIGHTED IMAGE, BRIGHT ON T2-WEIGHTED IMAGE, BRAIN STEM, NO MASS EFFECT

NONENHANCING
1. [CSF flow artifact]
2. Infarct/ischemic gliosis
3. Lupus erythematosus
4. Multiple sclerosis
5. Progressive multifocal leukoencephalopathy (PML)
6. Shearing injury (posterolateral upper brain stem)
7. Small low-grade glioma
8. Wallerian degeneration (eg, secondary to stroke or adrenoleukodystrophy)

ENHANCING
1. Acute multiple sclerosis
2. Small tumor (primary or metastasis)

Reference:
1. Bradley WG, Chapter 20, In: Stark DD, Bradley WG (eds): Magnetic Resonance Imaging. (ed 2) St. Louis: CV Mosby, 1992

Gamut M-21

DARK ON T1-WEIGHTED IMAGE, BRIGHT ON T2-WEIGHTED IMAGE, BRAIN STEM, MASS EFFECT

NONENHANCING
1. Early brain stem encephalitis
2. Low-grade glioma
3. Ramsay Hunt syndrome (retrograde spread of varicella virus)

ENHANCING
1. Abscess
2. Acute central pontine myelinolysis
3. Acute infarction
4. Acute tumefactive multiple sclerosis
5. Behcet's encephalitis
6. Brain stem encephalitis
7. Brain stem glioma
8. Ependymoblastoma (rare)
9. Ependymoma
10. Lymphoma_g
11. Metastasis
12. Perineural spread of squamous cell carcinoma
13. Primitive neuroectodermal tumor (PNET)

References:
1. Bradley WG, Chapter 20, In: Stark DD, Bradley WG (eds): Magnetic Resonance Imaging. (ed 2) St. Louis: CV Mosby, 1992
2. Hasso AN, et al., Chapter 27, In: Stark DD, Bradley WG (eds): Magnetic Resonance Imaging. (ed 2) St. Louis: CV Mosby, 1992

Gamut M-22

CEREBELLAR MASS

CHILD
1. Cystic astrocytoma
2. Medulloblastoma
3. Pilocytic astrocytoma

ADULT
1. Astrocytoma
2. Hemangioblastoma
3. Metastasis
4. Tumefactive multiple sclerosis

Reference:
1. Hasso AN, et al., Chapter 27, In: Stark DD, Bradley WG (edgs): Magnetic Resonance Imaging. (ed 2) St. Louis: CV Mosby, 1992

Gamut M-23

DARK ON T1-WEIGHTED IMAGE, BRIGHT ON T2-WEIGHTED IMAGE, ENHANCING CRANIAL NERVE

1. Neurinoma/schwannoma
2. Perineural spread of squamous cell carcinoma
3. Viral neuritis (eg, Bell's palsy)

Gamut M-24

DARK ON T1-WEIGHTED IMAGE, BRIGHT ON T2-WEIGHTED IMAGE, ENHANCING SELLA REGION LESION (See also Gamuts M-40, M-42, M-46, re: Other Sella Region Lesions)

Sellar/Parasellar Origin

1. Carotid aneurysm (cavernous, suprasellar)
2. Chordoma (rare)
3. Meningioma
4. Metastasis to pituitary
5. Mucocele of sphenoid sinus
6. Packing (fat or muscle) from previous transphenoidal hypophysectomy
7. Pituitary macroadenoma

Hypothalamic Origin

ENHANCING
1. Cystic craniopharyngioma
2. Germinoma (rare: ectopic pinealoma, multiple midline tumor syndrome)

NONENHANCING

1. Hamartoma of tuber cinereum (rare: may be isointense to brain)
2. Hypothalamic glioma

ENLARGED PITUITARY STALK

1. Histiocytosis X_g
2. Leptomeningeal carcinomatosis (esp. breast, lung)
3. Metastasis
4. Sarcoidosis

SMALL, NONENHANCING PITUITARY LESION

1. Fibrosis
2. Old hemorrhage
3. Pars intermedia cyst
4. [Partial volume cavernous carotid artery]
5. Pituitary microadenoma

Reference:

1. Hasso AN, Chapter 25, In: Stark DD, Bradley WG (eds): Magnetic Resonance Imaging. (ed 2) St. Louis: CV Mosby, 1992

Gamut M-25

DARK ON T1-WEIGHTED IMAGE, BRIGHT ON T2-WEIGHTED IMAGE, PINEAL REGION TUMOR

PINEAL ORIGIN

1. [Benign cystic pineal gland]
2. Pineoblastoma
3. Pineocytoma

GERM CELL ORIGIN

1. Choriocarcinoma (rare)
2. Embryonal carcinoma (rare)
3. Germinoma (common)
4. Teratoma

Reference:

1. Hasso AN, Chapter 25, In: Stark DD, Bradley WG (eds): Magnetic Resonance Imaging. (ed 2) St. Louis: CV Mosby, 1992

CSF INTENSITY LESION, PARENCHYMAL, NO MASS EFFECT

1. Cryptococcoma (early, in perivascular space)
2. Extrapontine myelinolysis
3. Macrocystic encephalomalacia (following stroke, trauma, bleed, surgery)
4. Marchiafava-Bignami disease (corpus callosum)
5. Mucopolysaccharidosis
6. [Perivascular space]
7. Porencephalic cyst

CSF INTENSITY, PARENCHYMAL, MASS EFFECT, NONENHANCING

1. Cryptococcoma
2. Cysticercus cyst (alive)
3. Echinococcal cyst (alive)
4. Parenchymal cyst

CSF INTENSITY, NONSPECIFIC LOCATION, MASS EFFECT, ENHANCING RIM OR NODULE

1. Cysticercus cyst (dead)
2. Cystic metastasis (eg, ovarian carcinoma)
3. Echinococcal cyst (dead)

Gamut M-29

CSF INTENSITY, BRAIN STEM

1. Central pontine myelinolysis
2. Infarct
3. Syringobulbia

Gamut M-30

CSF INTENSITY, POSTERIOR FOSSA

1. Arachnoid cyst
2. Cysticercosis
3. Dandy-Walker cyst or variant
4. Epidermoid
5. Mega cisterna magna
6. Trapped fourth ventricle

Gamut M-31

DARK ON T1-WEIGHTED IMAGE AND T2-WEIGHTED IMAGE, NONSPECIFIC LOCATION, NO MASS EFFECT

1. Calcified infection (TORCH: toxoplasma, rubella, CMV, herpes)
2. Chronic bleeding from cavernous angioma/venous angioma
3. Cysticercosis (old, calcified)
4. Hemorrhagic contusion (old)
5. Hemorrhagic shearing injury
6. Tuberculosis, treated (calcified)

M. MRI

Gamut M-32

DARK ON T1-WEIGHTED IMAGE AND T2-WEIGHTED IMAGE, NONSPECIFIC LOCATION, MASS EFFECT

1. Acute hemorrhage (intracellular deoxyhemoglobin)
2. Chloroma
3. Hemorrhagic leukoencephalopathy (autoimmune)
4. Short T2 metastases (mucinous adenocarcinoma of colon, melanoma, prostate, osteosarcoma)

Reference:

1. Bradley WG, Chapter 24, In: Stark DD, Bradley WG (eds): Magnetic Resonance Imaging. (ed 2) St. Louis: CV Mosby, 1992

Gamut M-33

DARK ON T1-WEIGHTED IMAGE AND T2-WEIGHTED IMAGE, CORTICAL, NO MASS EFFECT, NONENHANCING

1. Chronic hemorrhagic infarct (hemosiderin)
2. Superficial siderosis (following surgery or sub-arachnoid hemorrhage)

Gamut M-34

DARK ON T1-WEIGHTED IMAGE AND T2-WEIGHTED IMAGE, CORTICAL, NO MASS EFFECT, ENHANCING

1. Hemorrhagic cortical infarction (subacute)
2. Short T2 leptomeningeal metastases

Gamut M-35

DARK ON T1-WEIGHTED IMAGE AND T2-WEIGHTED IMAGE, CORTICAL, MASS EFFECT

1. Acute hemorrhagic contusion (deoxyhemoglobin)
2. Acute hemorrhagic cortical infarction

Gamut M-36

DARK ON T1-WEIGHTED IMAGE AND T2-WEIGHTED IMAGE, BASAL GANGLIA

1. Carbon monoxide poisoning
2. Ferrocalcinosis from hemorrhagic lacunar infarct
3. Hallervorden-Spatz disease
4. Idiopathic calcification
5. Ischemic-anoxic event in child (eg, near-drowning)
6. [Normal ferritin deposition (globus pallidus, putamen)]
7. Parkinson's plus (eg, Shy Drager, Progressive Supranuclear Palsy)

Reference:

1. Bradley WG, Chapter 24, In: Stark DD, Bradley WG (eds): Magnetic Resonance Imaging. (ed 2) St. Louis: CV Mosby, 1992

Gamut M-37

DARK ON T1-WEIGHTED IMAGE AND T2-WEIGHTED IMAGE, INTRAVASCULAR

1. Acute thrombosis (deoxyhemoglobin)
2. Calcific atherosclerosis
3. [Normal flow void]

Gamut M-38

DARK ON T1-WEIGHTED IMAGE AND T2-WEIGHTED IMAGE, BRAIN STEM

NORMAL STRUCTURES
1. [Corticospinal tracts]
2. [Medial lemnisci]
3. [Medial longitudinal fasciculi]

ABNORMAL
1. Acute hemorrhage (deoxyhemoglobin, eg, from hypertension)
2. Tortuous basilar artery

Reference:
1. Bradley WG, Chapter 20, In: Stark DD, Bradley WG (eds): Magnetic Resonance Imaging. (ed 2) St. Louis: CV Mosby, 1992

Gamut M-39

BRIGHT ON T1-WEIGHTED IMAGE AND T2-WEIGHTED IMAGE, NONSPECIFIC LOCATION

1. Cavernous angioma
2. Clotted aneurysm
3. [Flow artifact]
4. Late subacute hemorrhage (extracellular methemoglobin) (See B-39)
5. Venous infarction

Reference:
1. Bradley WG, Chapter 24, In: Stark DD, Bradley WG (eds): Magnetic Resonance Imaging. (ed 2) St. Louis: CV Mosby, 1992

Gamut M-40

BRIGHT ON T1-WEIGHTED IMAGE AND T2-WEIGHTED IMAGE, SELLA REGION

1. Clotted carotid aneurysm (late subacute hemorrhage)
2. Craniopharyngioma (proteinaceous, cystic)
3. Dermoid (proteinaceous, cystic)
4. [Diamagnetic susceptibility artifact]
5. Pituitary hemorrhage (late subacute hemorrhage, Sheehan's syndrome, Simmonds' syndrome, following bromocryptine therapy)
6. Rathke's cleft cyst

Reference:

1. Hasso AN, et al., Chapter 25, In: Stark DD, Bradley WG (eds): Magnetic Resonance Imaging. (ed 2) St. Louis: CV Mosby, 1992

Gamut M-41

BRIGHT ON T1-WEIGHTED IMAGE, DARK ON T2-WEIGHTED IMAGE, NONSPECIFIC LOCATION

1. Calcification (eg, basal ganglia)
2. Clotted aneurysm (early subacute hemorrhage)
3. Dermoid
4. Early subacute hemorrhage (See B-39) (intracellular methemoglobin)
5. [Flow artifact]
6. Lipoma
7. "White" epidermoid (liquid triglyceride)

Reference:

1. Bradley WG, Chapter 24, In: Stark DD, Bradley WG (eds): Magnetic Resonance Imaging. (ed 2) St. Louis: CV Mosby, 1992

Gamut M-42

BRIGHT ON T1-WEIGHTED IMAGE, DARK ON T2-WEIGHTED IMAGE, SELLA REGION

1. Dermoid (fatty)
2. Early subacute pituitary hemorrhage (intracellular methemoglobin)
3. Ectopic posterior pituitary (following distal stalk transection)
4. Lipoma
5. [Normal posterior lobe of pituitary]
6. "White" epidermoid

Gamut M-43

SIGNAL VOID, NONSPECIFIC LOCATION

1. Aneurysm
2. Arteriovenous malformation (AVM)
3. Bone fragment (posttrauma)
4. Collateral vessels (eg, in basal ganglia due to moya-moya)
5. Congenital AIDS (calcification)
6. Dense calcification (previous bleed, tumor)
7. Densely calcified old infection (TORCH-toxoplasmosis, rubella, CMV, herpes; syphilis, cysticercosis)
8. Enlarged medullary vein
9. [Normal vessel (artery, dural sinus)]
10. Pneumocephalus
11. Shunt tube
12. Tuberculosis (treated)
13. Venous angioma

Gamut M-44

SIGNAL VOID, SUBEPENDYMAL

1. Arteriovenous malformation (AVM)
2. Calcified hamartomas (tuberous sclerosis)
3. Shunt tube
4. Venous angioma

Gamut M-45

SIGNAL VOID, BRAIN STEM

1. Arteriovenous malformation (AVM)
2. Ectatic, tortuous vertebral or basilar artery

Gamut M-46

SIGNAL VOID, SELLA REGION

1. Basilar tip aneurysm
2. Carotid-cavernous fistula
3. Cavernous or supraclinoid carotid aneurysm
4. Meningioma (densely calcified)
5. [Metallic artifact (from clipped aneurysm)]
5. Pneumatized posterior clinoid

Gamut M-47

SMALL VENTRICLES, SMALL SULCI

1. Diffuse brain edema
2. [Normal variant]
3. Pseudotumor cerebri

Gamut M-48

ENLARGED VENTRICLES, SMALL SULCI

1. Central atrophy (due to deep white matter ischemia, near drowning [or other ischemia-anoxia], multiple sclerosis)
2. Communicating hydrocephalus (See M-48A)
3. Culpocephaly (dilated occipital horns only)
4. Obstructive hydrocephalus (See M-48B)

Subgamut M-48A

CAUSES OF COMMUNICATING HYDROCEPHALUS (OBSTRUCTION BETWEEN OUTLET FORAMINA OF FOURTH VENTRICLE AND ARACHNOID VILLI) (See Gamut B-48)

1. Dural sinus/cortical venous thrombosis
2. Idiopathic ("normal pressure hydrocephalus")
3. Leptomeningeal carcinomatosis (metastatic breast carcinoma [adults], medulloblastoma [children], leukemia, lymphoma)
4. Meningitis
5. Subarachnoid hemorrhage

Reference:
1. Bradley WG, Chapter 28, In: Stark DD, Bradley WG (eds): Magnetic Resonance Imaging. (ed 2) St. Louis: CV Mosby, 1992

Subgamut M-48B

CAUSES OF OBSTRUCTIVE HYDROCEPHALUS (OBSTRUCTION PROXIMAL TO FORAMINA OF LUSCHKA AND MAGENDIE) (See Gamut B-48)

1. Congenital aqueductal stenosis
2. Encephalitis (at foramen of Monro, aqueduct, fourth ventricle)
3. Inflammation/ventriculitis (at foramen of Monro, aqueduct)
4. Tumefactive multiple sclerosis (at foramen of Monro, aqueduct, fourth ventricle)
5. Tumor (at foramen of Monro, aqueduct, fourth ventricle, cerebellopontine angle [eg, large acoustic neurinoma])

Reference:
1. Bradley WG, Chapter 28, In: Stark DD, Bradley WG (eds): Magnetic Resonance Imaging. (ed 2) St. Louis: CV Mosby, 1992

Gamut M-49

ENLARGED VENTRICLES, ENLARGED SULCI

1. Alcoholism
2. Anorexia nervosa
3. Atrophy (due to AIDS, dehydration, multiple sclerosis, radiation therapy, chemotherapy, trauma, postinfectious, global ischemia, Alzheimer's disease)
4. Catabolic steroids
5. Creutzfeldt-Jakob disease
6. Cushing's disease

7. External hydrocephalus (communicating hydrocephalus in child under two years of age)
8. Kwashiorkor
9. Starvation

Reference:

1. Bradley WG, Chapter 28, In: Stark DD, Bradley WG (eds): Magnetic Resonance Imaging. (ed 2) St. Louis: CV Mosby, 1992

Gamut M-50

ABNORMAL VENTRICULAR CONFIGURATION

1. Agenesis of corpus callosum (high-riding third ventricle between lateral ventricles)
2. Alobar and semilobar holoprosencephaly (single ventricle)
3. Asymmetry of lateral ventricles (normal variant, obstruction of one foramen of Monro, inflammation, hemiatrophy [Davidoff-Dyke])
4. Cavum of the velum interpositum (triangular CSF space separating posterior lateral ventricular bodies)
5. Cavum septum pellucidum and vergae (separation of lateral ventricles)
6. Hemimegalencephaly (single, enlarged, misshapen lateral ventricle with surrounding heterotopic gray matter)
7. Periventricular leukomalacia (enlarged, irregular lateral ventricles)
8. Schizencephaly (lateral ventricular wall tethered laterally by gray matter-lined cleft)

Reference:

1. Zimmerman RA, Chapter 31, In: Stark DD, Bradley WG (eds): Magnetic Resonance Imaging. (ed 2) St. Louis: CV Mosby, 1992

Gamut M-51

INTRAVENTRICULAR MASS, CSF INTENSITY

1. Arachnoid cyst
2. Cysticercosis
3. Dandy-Walker cyst or variant (fourth ventricle)

Gamut M-52

INTRAVENTRICULAR MASS, DARK ON T1-WEIGHTED IMAGE, BRIGHT ON T2-WEIGHTED IMAGE, NONENHANCING

1. "Black" epidermoid (solid cholesterol/cholesterin)
2. Colloid cyst (third ventricle)
3. Neuroepithelial cyst (choroid plexus)

Gamut M-53

INTRAVENTRICULAR MASS, DARK ON T1-WEIGHTED IMAGE, BRIGHT ON T2-WEIGHTED IMAGE, ENHANCING

1. Colloid cyst
2. Choroid plexus papilloma/carcinoma
3. Choroidal metastasis (esp, lung, colon, breast, melanoma)
4. Ependymoma
5. Intraventricular glioma/astrocytoma
6. Intraventricular meningioma
7. Intraventricular spread of high-grade glioma
8. Subependymoma (rare, usually infratentorial)

References:
1. Pomeranz SJ, Gamuts and Pearls in MRI. Richmond: Wm Byrd Press, 1990
2. Hasso AN, et al., Chapter 25, In: Stark DD, Bradley WG (eds): Magnetic Resonance Imaging. (ed 2) St. Louis: CV Mosby, 1992

Gamut M-54

INTRAVENTRICULAR MASS, DARK ON T1-WEIGHTED IMAGE AND T2-WEIGHTED IMAGE

1. Acute hematoma (deoxyhemoglobin)
2. Calcified glomus of choroid plexus
3. Densely calcified meningioma

Gamut M-55

INTRAVENTRICULAR MASS, BRIGHT ON T1-WEIGHTED IMAGE

DARK ON T2-WEIGHTED IMAGE
1. Dermoid
2. Early subacute hemorrhage (intracellular methemoglobin)
3. Lipoma
4. Pantopaque
5. Xanthogranuloma of choroid plexus

BRIGHT ON T2-WEIGHTED IMAGE
1. Late subacute hemorrhage (extracellular methemoglobin)

Gamut M-56

INTRAVENTRICULAR SIGNAL VOID

1. Hyperdynamic CSF flow (communicating hydrocephalus, shunt-responsive normal pressure hydrocephalus [NPH])
2. [Normal CSF flow (near aqueduct and foramen of Monro)]
3. Pneumocephalus (postoperative, posttraumatic)
4. Vein of Galen "aneurysm" (posterior third ventricle)

Reference:
1. Bradley WG, Chapter 28, In: Stark DD, Bradley WG (eds): Magnetic Resonance Imaging. (ed 2) St. Louis: CV Mosby, 1992

Gamut M-57

SUBARACHNOID SPACE, ISOINTENSE TO BRAIN

1. Acute subarachnoid hemorrhage (protein effect)
2. [CSF flow (flow related enhancement, even echo rephasing/gradient moment nulling)]
3. Meningitis

Reference:
1. Bradley WG, Chapters 11 and 24, In: Stark DD, Bradley WG (eds): Magnetic Resonance Imaging. (ed 2) St. Louis: CV Mosby, 1992

Gamut M-58

SUBARACHNOID SPACE, HYPERINTENSE TO BRAIN ON T1-WEIGHTED IMAGE AND PROTON DENSITY-WEIGHTED IMAGE

1. [CSF flow (flow-related enhancement)]
2. Dermoid
3. Lipoma (eg, cerebellopontine angle)
4. Pantopaque
5. Subacute subarachnoid thrombus (methemoglobin)
6. White epidermoid

Gamut M-59

SUBARACHNOID SPACE, ISOINTENSE TO CSF

1. Arachnoid cyst (in middle fossa, posterior fossa, interhemispheric, or suprasellar) (post-trauma/infection, or associated with acoustic neurinoma)
2. Cysticercosis (basilar racemose form)

Gamut M-60

SUBARACHNOID SPACE, SIGNAL VOID

1. [Normal CSF flow]
2. [Normal flow in artery]
3. [Juxta-arterial CSF dephasing]
4. [Postoperative metallic (clip) artifact]

Reference:
1. Bradley WG, Chapters 11 and 24, In: Stark DD, Bradley WG (eds): Magnetic Resonance Imaging. (ed 2) St. Louis: CV Mosby, 1992

Gamut M-61

MASS IN THE CEREBELLOPONTINE ANGLE CISTERN

Enhancing

COMMON
1. Acoustic neurinoma/schwannoma
2. Meningioma
3. Trigeminal schwannoma (may have "dumbbell" shape with second mass in cavernous sinus)

UNCOMMON
1. Aneurysm of vertebral artery
2. Chordoma
3. Exophytic ependymoma or brain stem glioma
4. Glomus tumor (jugulare, tympanicum, vagale)

Nonenhancing

1. Arachnoid cyst
2. Epidermoid
3. Lipoma (may simulate enhanced acoustic neurinoma)

Reference:
1. Hasso AN, et al. Chapter 26, In: Stark DD, Bradley WG (eds): Magnetic Resonance Imaging. (ed 2) St. Louis: CV Mosby, 1992

FOCAL LEPTOMENINGEAL ENHANCEMENT

1. Leptomeningeal carcinomatosis (eg, breast, lung, melanoma)
2. Lymphoma$_g$
3. Meningitis
4. Postoperative scarring
5. Sarcoidosis
6. Subjacent acute infarction (pial collaterals)

DIFFUSE LEPTOMENINGEAL ENHANCEMENT

1. Leptomeningeal carcinomatosis (eg, breast, lung, melanoma)
2. Meningitis (bacterial [common]; fungal and viral [rare])
3. Post subarachnoid hemorrhage
4. Post surgery
5. Post trauma

PACHYMENINGEAL (DURAL) NONENHANCING LESION

1. Dense calcification (black)
2. Densely calcified meningioma
3. Ossification (black rim, fatty center)

Gamut M-65

PACHYMENINGEAL (DURAL) ENHANCING LESION

1. Benign meningeal fibrosis (following shunt, subarachnoid hemorrhage, or surgery)
2. Dural metastasis (eg, neuroblastoma)
3. Local tumor spread (eg, from glioblastoma)
4. Meningioma
5. [Normal (especially at high field with high-dose gadolinium)]

Gamut M-66

EXTRAAXIAL FLUID COLLECTION, CSF INTENSITY

1. Arachnoid cyst
2. Benign subdural effusions (in neonatal meningitis)
3. Chronic subdural hematoma (subdural hygroma)
4. Cysticercosis
5. External hydrocephalus (under age 2)
6. Posttraumatic arachnoid rent

Gamut M-67

EXTRAAXIAL FLUID COLLECTION, DARK ON T1-WEIGHTED IMAGE

BRIGHT ON T2-WEIGHTED IMAGE
1. Chronic subdural/epidural hematoma
2. Subdural/epidural empyema

DARK ON T2-WEIGHTED IMAGE
1. Acute subdural/epidural hematoma
2. Extraaxial air (postoperative, posttraumatic)

Reference:
1. Bradley WG, Chapter 24, In: Stark DD, Bradley WG (eds): Magnetic Resonance Imaging. (ed 2) St. Louis: CV Mosby, 1992

Gamut M-68

EXTRAAXIAL FLUID COLLECTION, BRIGHT ON T1-WEIGHTED IMAGE

BRIGHT ON T2-WEIGHTED IMAGE
1. Late subacute subdural/epidural hematoma (extracellular methemoglobin)

DARK ON T2-WEIGHTED IMAGE
1. Early subacute subdural/epidural hematoma (intracellular methemoglobin)

Reference:
1. Bradley WG, Chapter 24, In: Stark DD, Bradley WG (eds): Magnetic Resonance Imaging. (ed 2) St. Louis: CV Mosby, 1992

Gamut M-69

EXTRAAXIAL MASS, NONENHANCING

1. Arachnoid cyst
2. Epidermoid

Gamut M-70

EXTRAAXIAL MASS, ENHANCING

1. Dural metastasis
2. Hemangiopericytoma of meninges (angioblastic meningioma-rare)
3. Meningioma
4. Neurinoma/schwannoma of cranial nerve (eg, acoustic)
5. Upper cervical neurofibroma extending through foramen magnum

Reference:
1. Hasso AN, et al., Chapters 26 and 27, In: Stark DD, Bradley WG (eds): Magnetic Resonance Imaging. (ed 2) St. Louis: CV Mosby, 1992

Gamut M-71

EXTRACRANIAL MASS, CSF INTENSITY

1. Encephalocele
2. Meningocele
3. Postoperative CSF leak (pseudomeningocele)

Gamut M-72

EXTRACRANIAL MASS, DARK ON T1-WEIGHTED IMAGE

1. Acute cephalohematoma (dark on T2-weighted image) (intracellular deoxyhemoglobin)
2. Chronic cephalohematoma (bright on T2-weighted image)
3. Hemangioma
4. Lymphangioma
5. Sebaceous cyst

Gamut M-73

EXTRACRANIAL MASS, BRIGHT ON T1-WEIGHTED IMAGE

1. Lipoma
2. Subacute cephalohematoma (methemoglobin)

Gamut M-74

LESION OF THE GLOBE

Bright on T2-Weighted Image

COMMON
1. Choroidal metastasis (breast, lung)
2. Retinal detachment

UNCOMMON
1. Choroidal hemangioma
2. Retinal cyst

Dark on T2-Weighted Image

COMMON
1. Primary or metastatic melanoma
2. Retinoblastoma (child)

UNCOMMON
1. Astrocytic hamartoma
2. Benign melanocytoma
3. Endophthalmitis
4. Glass prosthesis
5. Phthisis bulbi
6. Pseudotumor
7. Sarcoidosis

Reference:
1. Atlas SW, Chapter 30, In: Stark DD, Bradley WG (eds): Magnetic Resonance Imaging. (ed 2) St. Louis: CV Mosby, 1992

Gamut M-75

OPTIC NERVE/NERVE SHEATH LESION

INTERMEDIATE SIGNAL ON T2-WEIGHTED IMAGE (COMMON)

1. Optic nerve glioma
2. Optic nerve sheath meningioma
3. Optic neuritis

HIGH SIGNAL ON T2-WEIGHTED IMAGE (UNCOMMON)

1. Dural ectasia

Reference:
1. Atlas SW, Chapter 30, In: Stark DD, Bradley WG (eds): Magnetic Resonance Imaging. (ed 2) St. Louis: CV Mosby, 1992

Gamut M-76

RETROBULBAR MASS

Isointense to Fat on T2-Weighted Image

COMMON

1. Dermoid
2. Lacrimal gland tumors (See M-78)
3. Lymphoma$_g$
4. Optic nerve sheath meningioma
5. Pseudotumor
6. Thyroid orbitopathy (Graves' disease)

UNCOMMON

1. Amyloid
2. Arteriovenous malformation (AVM)

3. Lipoma
4. Myeloma
5. Sarcoidosis

Brighter than Fat on T2-Weighted Image

COMMON

1. Cavernous hemangioma
2. Dermoid
3. Extraconal meningioma
4. Hematoma following trauma or surgery
5. Lacrimal gland tumors (See M-78)
6. Plexiform neurofibroma
7. Schwannoma

UNCOMMON

1. Bacterial infection
2. Brown tumor (hyperparathyroidism)
3. Histiocytosis X_g
4. Lymphangioma
5. Metastases (children: neuroblastoma, leukemia, Ewing's sarcoma; adults: carcinoma of the breast or lung)

Reference:

1. Atlas SW, Chapter 30, In: Stark DD, Bradley WG (eds): Magnetic Resonance Imaging. (ed 2) St. Louis: CV Mosby, 1992

Gamut M-77

EXTRAOCULAR MUSCLE ENLARGEMENT

ISOINTENSE TO FAT ON T2-WEIGHTED IMAGE
1. Acromegaly
2. Infection
3. Pseudotumor
4. Sarcoidosis
5. Thyroid orbitopathy, bilateral (Graves' disease)
6. Venous obstruction

BRIGHTER THAN FAT ON T2-WEIGHTED IMAGE
1. Bacterial infection (from adjacent sinus infection)
2. Carotid-cavernous fistula (traumatic; dural AVM)
3. Hematoma
4. Leukemia
5. Lymphangioma
6. Lymphoma$_g$
7. Metastases (breast, lung)
8. Rhabdomyosarcoma (child)
9. Trauma

Reference:
1. Atlas SW, Chapter 30, In: Stark DD, Bradley WG (eds): Magnetic Resonance Imaging. (ed 2) St. Louis: CV Mosby, 1992

Gamut M-78

LATERAL EXTRACONAL LESION

BRIGHT ON T2-WEIGHTED IMAGE
1. Inflammation of lacrimal gland (eg, sarcoidosis - generally bilateral)
2. Metastatic disease
3. Primary tumor of lacrimal gland (benign mixed tumor, adenoid cystic carcinoma, lymphoma$_g$ - usually bilateral)

DARK ON T2-WEIGHTED IMAGE

1. Extraconal meningioma
2. [Normal lacrimal gland]

Reference:

1. Atlas SW, Chapter 30, In: Stark DD, Bradley WG (eds): Magnetic
   Resonance Imaging. (ed 2) St. Louis: CV Mosby, 1992

Gamut M-79

ENLARGED SUPERIOR OPHTHALMIC VEIN

1. Carotid-cavernous fistula (traumatic; dural AVM)
2. [Normal variant]
3. Orbital apex mass
4. Pseudotumor
5. Thyroid orbitopathy (Graves' disease)
6. Varix, varicocele, venous angioma

Reference:

1. Atlas SW, Chapter 30, In: Stark DD, Bradley WG (eds): Magnetic
   Resonance Imaging. (ed 2) St. Louis: CV Mosby, 1992

Gamut M-80

THROMBOSIS OF SUPERIOR OPHTHALMIC VEIN

1. Adjacent orbital infection
2. Cavernous sinus thrombosis (secondary to tumor,
   inflammation, trauma)
3. Dural AVM
4. Varix

Reference:

1. Atlas SW, Chapter 30, In: Stark DD, Bradley WG (eds): Magnetic
   Resonance Imaging. (ed 2) St. Louis: CV Mosby, 1992

Gamut M-81

ORBITAL WALL LESION

HYPOINTENSE ON T2-WEIGHTED IMAGE
1. Chondrosarcoma
2. Fibrous dysplasia
3. Histiocytosis X_g
4. Hyperostosis due to meningioma
5. Osteoblastic osteosarcoma
6. Osteoma

HYPERINTENSE ON T2-WEIGHTED IMAGE
1. Cystic chondrosarcoma
2. Epidermoid
3. Ewing's sarcoma (child)
4. Frontonasal encephalocele
5. Giant cell granuloma
6. Giant cell tumor
7. Infection
8. Lymphangioma
9. Lymphoma$_g$
10. Metastatic disease
11. Mucocele
12. Neuroblastoma (child)

References:
1. Pomeranz SJ, Gamuts and Pearls in MRI. Richmond: Wm Byrd Press, 1990
2. Atlas SW, Chapter 30, In: Stark DD, Bradley WG (eds): Magnetic Resonance Imaging. (ed 2) St. Louis: CV Mosby, 1992

Gamut M-82

SINONASAL MASS WITHOUT BONE CHANGES, BRIGHT ON T2-WEIGHTED IMAGE

COMMON
1. Acute infection
2. Mucous retention cyst
3. Polyp

UNCOMMON
1. Epidermoid
2. Lymphoma_g

Reference:
1. Som PM, Curtin HD, Chapter 35, In: Stark DD, Bradley WG (eds): Magnetic Resonance Imaging. (ed 2) St. Louis: CV Mosby, 1992

Gamut M-83

SINONASAL MASS WITHOUT BONE CHANGES, DARK ON T2-WEIGHTED IMAGE

1. Acute hemorrhage
2. Air
3. Dentigerous cyst
4. Dried secretions
5. Mycetoma (eg, aspergillosis)
6. Osteoma
7. Sinolith
8. Undescended maxillary tooth

Gamut M-84

SINONASAL MASS WITH BONY REMODELING WITHOUT EROSION

COMMON

1. Mucocele
2. Pyomucocele

UNCOMMON

1. Esthesioneuroblastoma
2. Histiocytic lymphoma
3. Inverting papilloma
4. Most minor salivary gland tumors
5. Neurinomas
6. Some sarcomas

Reference:

1. Som PM, Curtin HD, Chapter 35, In: Stark DD, Bradley WG (eds): Magnetic Resonance Imaging. (ed 2) St. Louis: CV Mosby, 1992

Gamut M-85

SINONASAL MASS WITH BONY EROSION

COMMON

1. Adenoid cystic carcinoma (perineural extension)
2. Angiofibroma (boys)
3. Squamous cell carcinoma (adults)

UNCOMMON

1. Adenocarcinoma
2. Extracranial meningioma
3. High-grade minor salivary gland carcinoma

Reference:

1. Som PM, Curtin HD, Chapter 35, In: Stark DD, Bradley WG (eds): Magnetic Resonance Imaging. (ed 2) St. Louis: CV Mosby, 1992

VASCULAR SINONASAL MASS WITH FLOW VOIDS

COMMON
1. Juvenile angiofibroma (boys)
2. Metastatic disease (renal, thyroid)

UNCOMMON
1. Hemangioma
2. Hemangiopericytoma

Reference:
1. Som PM, Curtin HD, Chapter 35, In: Stark DD, Bradley WG (eds): Magnetic Resonance Imaging. (ed 2) St. Louis: CV Mosby, 1992

FIBRO-OSSEOUS LESION OF A PARANASAL SINUS

DARK ON T2-WEIGHTED IMAGE
1. Fibrous dysplasia
2. Nonossifying fibroma
3. Ossifying fibroma
4. Osteoma

BRIGHT ON T2-WEIGHTED IMAGE
1. Osteoblastoma
2. Osteosarcoma

Reference:
1. Som PM, Curtin HD, Chapter 35, In: Stark DD, Bradley WG (eds): Magnetic Resonance Imaging. (ed 2) St. Louis: CV Mosby, 1992

Gamut M-88

SKULL BASE LESION

COMMON

Bright on T2-Weighted Image
1. Chondroma, osteochondroma
2. Epidermoid
3. Ewing's sarcoma (child)
4. Hemangioma/vascular hamartoma of facial nerve
5. Osseous metastasis
6. Paraganglioma (glomus tympanicum)
7. Schwannoma of fifth and eighth cranial nerves
8. Squamous cell carcinoma extending through basal foramina

Dark on T2-Weighted Image
1. Histiocytosis X_g (child)
2. Meningioma

UNCOMMON

Bright on T2-Weighted Image
1. Aneurysmal bone cyst
2. Chordoma
3. Cholesterol granuloma
4. Fibrosarcoma (following Paget's disease, fibrous dysplasia, osteomyelitis, radiation therapy)
5. Giant cell tumor (young adults)
6. Petrous apicitis
7. Pituitary macroadenoma
8. Plasmacytoma
9. Schwannoma of cranial nerves VII and IX-XII

Reference:
1. Hasso AN, et al., Chapter 27, In: Stark DD, Bradley WG (eds): Magnetic Resonance Imaging. (ed 2) St. Louis: CV Mosby, 1992

Gamut M-89

NASOPHARYNGEAL MASS

COMMON
1. Adenoiditis
2. Juvenile angiofibroma
3. Non-Hodgkin's lymphoma
4. Squamous cell carcinoma
5. Thornwaldt cyst (midline posterior nasopharyngeal recess)

UNCOMMON
1. Adenocarcinoma
2. Adenoid cystic carcinoma (perineural spread)
3. Malignant otitis externa extending medially
4. Mucormycosis

Reference:
1. Teresi LM, et al, Chapter 37, In: Stark DD, Bradley WG (eds): Magnetic Resonance Imaging. (ed 2) St. Louis: CV Mosby, 1992

Gamut M-90

PRESTYLOID PHARYNGEAL MASS

COMMON
1. Benign mixed tumor arising from accessory salivary gland
2. Deep lobe parotid tumor (benign mixed tumor [pleomorphic adenoma])

UNCOMMON
1. Adenocarcinoma
2. Atypical lymphoepithelial lesions
3. Branchial cleft cyst
4. Lipoma

Reference:
1. Kramer LA, Mafee MF, Chapter 37, In: Stark DD, Bradley WG (eds): Magnetic Resonance Imaging. (ed 2) St. Louis: CV Mosby, 1992

Gamut M-91

POSTSTYLOID PHARYNGEAL MASS

COMMON
1. Benign mixed tumor arising from accessory salivary tissue (pleomorphic adenoma)
2. Enlarged lateral retropharyngeal lymph node
3. Schwannoma/neurofibroma

UNCOMMON
1. Paraganglioma

Reference:
1. Kramer LA, Mafee MF, Chapter 37, In: Stark DD, Bradley WG (eds): Magnetic Resonance Imaging. (ed 2) St. Louis: CV Mosby, 1992

Gamut M-92

TONGUE/ORAL CAVITY MASS

COMMON
1. Schwannoma
2. Squamous cell carcinoma

UNCOMMON
1. Adenocarcinoma
2. Amyloid
3. Bacterial cellulitis/abscess (Vincent's angina)

4. Dermoid
5. Hemangioma
6. Lingual thyroid
7. Lymphoid hyperplasia of lingual tonsil
8. Lymphoma$_g$
9. Metastasis
10. Minor salivary gland malignancy (adenoid cystic carcinoma, mucoepidermoid carcinoma, adenocarcinoma)
11. Ranula
12. Thyroglossal duct cyst

Reference:
1. Teresi LM, et al, Chapter 36, In: Stark DD, Bradley WG (eds): Magnetic Resonance Imaging. (ed 2) St. Louis: CV Mosby, 1992

Gamut M-93

SALIVARY GLAND LESION

COMMON

Intermediate on T2-Weighted Image
1. Benign mixed tumors (pleomorphic adenomas [most common in superficial lobe of parotid])
2. Epidemic parotitis (mumps)
3. Intraparotid lymphadenopathy (See M-93A)
4. Lipoma
5. Mucoepidermoid carcinoma (low grade)
6. Sarcoidosis
7. Schwannoma/neurofibroma
8. Systemic lymphoma$_g$

Bright on T2-Weighted Image
1. Branchial cleft cyst
2. Cystic hygroma (lymphangioma)
3. Hemangioma
4. Parotid cysts (AIDS)
5. Ranula

UNCOMMON

1. Actinomycosis
2. Acute suppurative sialoadenitis
3. Adenocarcinoma
4. Adenoid cystic carcinoma
5. Chronic recurrent sialoadenitis
6. Chronic sialectasis
7. High-grade mucoepidermoid carcinoma (more often in deep lobe of parotid)
8. Lymphoepithelial sialoadenopathy
9. Metastatic disease (from cutaneous squamous cell carcinoma, melanoma, lung, breast, kidney)
10. Primary lymphoma$_g$
11. Sarcoma
12. Sialolithiasis
13. Squamous cell carcinoma
14. Syphilis
15. Tuberculosis
16. Undifferentiated carcinoma

Reference:
1. Kramer LA, Mafee MF, Chapter 37, In: Stark DD, Bradley WG (eds): Magnetic Resonance Imaging. (ed 2) St. Louis: CV Mosby, 1992

Subgamut M-93A

CAUSES OF INTRAPAROTID LYMPHADENOPATHY

1. AIDS
2. Chronic autoimmune sialoadenitis (Sjögren's syndrome)
3. Lymphadenitis
4. Metastatic disease
5. Sarcoidosis
6. Toxoplasmosis
7. Tuberculosis

Reference:
1. Kramer LA, Mafee MF, Chapter 37, In: Stark DD, Bradley WG (eds): Magnetic Resonance Imaging. (ed 2) St. Louis: CV Mosby, 1992

Gamut M-94

MASS OF THE HYPOPHARYNX OR LARYNX

COMMON
1. Polyp (papilloma)
2. Squamous cell carcinoma

UNCOMMON
1. Adenocarcinoma
2. Adenoma
3. Amyloidosis
4. Basal cell carcinoma
5. Chondroma
6. Hemangioma
7. Kaposi's sarcoma
8. Lymphoma$_g$
9. Neurofibroma
10. Plasmacytoma
11. Posttraumatic changes
12. Wegener's granulomatosis

Reference:
1. Vogl TJ, Chapter 38, In: Stark DD, Bradley WG (eds): Magnetic Resonance Imaging. (ed 2) St. Louis: CV Mosby, 1992

Gamut M-95

MASS IN THE NECK

COMMON

Intermediate on T2-Weighted Image
1. Goiter
2. Jugular thrombophlebitis (acute, early subacute)
3. Lipoma
4. Lymphadenopathy (infectious, metastatic disease, lymphoma$_g$)
5. Thyroid adenoma
6. Thyroid carcinoma

Bright on T2-Weighted Image
1. Abscess
2. Hemangioma
3. Jugular thrombophlebitis (late subacute, chronic)
4. Thyroglossal duct cyst (midline)

UNCOMMON

Intermediate on T2-Weighted Image
1. Neuroblastoma (child)
2. Plexiform neurofibroma
3. Teratoma (fatty, solid)

Bright on T2-Weighted Image
1. Colloid cyst of thyroid gland
2. Hygroma
3. Laryngocele
4. Lymphocele
5. Paraganglioma (glomus caroticum)
6. Schwannoma
7. Second branchial cleft cyst (lateral)
8. Teratoma (cystic)
9. Thymic cyst
10. Tracheoesophageal cyst

Reference:
1. Vogl TJ, Chapter 38, In: Stark DD, Bradley WG (eds): Magnetic Resonance Imaging. (ed 2) St. Louis: CV Mosby, 1992

Gamut M-96

FOCAL VERTEBRAL BODY ABNORMALITY WITH DECREASED SIGNAL ON T1-WEIGHTED IMAGE AND INCREASED SIGNAL ON T2-WEIGHTED IMAGE

1. Acute fracture
2. [Flow artifact from aorta or iliac arteries]
3. GCSF (granulocyte colony stimulating factor) therapy
4. Infection (from osteomyelitis or diskitis)
5. Marrow replacement
6. Multiple myeloma
7. Osseous metastasis
8. Primary bone tumor (eg, Ewing's, lymphoma, osteosarcoma)
9. Type I degenerative endplate changes

Reference:
1. Shoukimas GM: Chapter 41, In: Stark DD, Bradley WG (eds): Magnetic Resonance Imaging. (ed 2) St. Louis: CV Mosby, 1992

3. Cord edema (eg, due to herniated disk)
4. [CSF motion artifact]
5. Devic's syndrome (demyelination of cord and optic neuritis)
6. Gliosis
7. Multiple sclerosis
8. Small glioma
9. Small nonhemorrhagic contusion
10. Subacute infarct
11. [Truncation artifact]

Reference:
1. Houghton V, et al: Chapter 40, In: Stark DD, Bradley WG (eds): Magnetic Resonance Imaging. (ed 2) St. Louis: CV Mosby, 1992

Gamut M-101

INTRAMEDULLARY LESION, DARK ON T1-WEIGHTED IMAGE, BRIGHT ON T2-WEIGHTED IMAGE, WITH MASS EFFECT

COMMON
1. Acute contusion
2. Acute disseminated encephalomyelitis (ADEM)
3. Astrocytoma
4. Ependymoma
5. Hemangioblastoma
6. Leptomeningeal carcinomatosis (eg, breast)
7. Myelitis

UNCOMMON
1. Acute infarct
2. Acute tumefactive multiple sclerosis
3. Drop metastasis down central canal (eg, medulloblastoma)
4. Lymphoma
5. Radiation necrosis
6. Spinal meningitis

References:

1. Houghton V, et al: Chapter 40, In: Stark DD, Bradley WG (eds): Magnetic Resonance Imaging. (ed 2) St. Louis: CV Mosby, 1992
2. Shoukimas GM: Chapter 41, In: Stark DD, Bradley WG (eds): Magnetic Resonance Imaging. (ed 2) St. Louis: CV Mosby, 1992

Gamut M-102

INTRAMEDULLARY LESION, DARK ON T1 AND T2-WEIGHTED IMAGES, WITH MASS EFFECT

1. Focal calcification
2. Hemosiderin from old bleed (eg, from cavernous angioma or AVM)
3. [Metallic artifact from previous surgery]
4. Osseous spur in diastematomyelia

Gamut M-103

INTRAMEDULLARY LESION, BRIGHT ON T1-WEIGHTED IMAGE

BRIGHT ON T2-WEIGHTED IMAGE

1. Late subacute hematomyelia (extracellular met-hemoglobin from tumor, AVM, trauma)
2. Proteinaceous cyst (eg, from tumor)

DARK ON T2-WEIGHTED IMAGE

1. Early subacute hematomyelia (intracellular met-hemoglobin from tumor, AVM, trauma)

UNCOMMON

1. Choroid plexus carcinoma
2. Pineoblastoma
3. Pineocytoma
4. Teratoma

Non-CNS Sources

1. Metastatic carcinoma (esp. breast, lung)
2. Metastatic lymphoma
3. Metastatic melanoma

Reference:

1. Shoukimas GM: Chapter 41, In: Stark DD, Bradley WG (eds): Magnetic Resonance Imaging. (ed 2) St. Louis: CV Mosby, 1992

Gamut M-107

EXTRAMEDULLARY, INTRADURAL LESION, BRIGHT ON T1-WEIGHTED IMAGE, DARK ON T2-WEIGHTED IMAGE

1. Dermoid (fatty)
2. Fatty filum
3. Lipoma
4. Pantopaque
5. White epidermoid

Reference:

1. Shoukimas GM: Chapter 41, In: Stark DD, Bradley WG (eds): Magnetic Resonance Imaging. (ed 2) St. Louis: CV Mosby, 1992

Gamut M-108

EXTRAMEDULLARY, INTRADURAL SIGNAL VOID

1. Arteriovenous malformation
2. [CSF flow artifact]
3. [Metallic artifact]

Gamut M-109

EXTRADURAL LESION WITH NORMAL ADJACENT BONE (See Gamut S-59)

At Level of Disk Only

1. Disk bulge
2. Disk extrusion
3. Disk protrusion
4. Epidural scar (eg, after disk surgery)
5. Marginal osteophyte

Not Necessarily at Level of Disk

1. Arachnoid cyst
2. Conjoined root sleeve
3. Epidural abscess
4. Epidural granuloma (eg, tuberculous, fungal, sarcoid, schistosomal)
5. Epidural hematoma
6. Epidural lipomatosis (obesity, steroid therapy, Cushing S.)
7. Epidural metastasis
8. Extruded or sequestered disk
9. Lipoma (spinal dysraphism)
10. Lymphoma$_g$

Glossary

ANEMIA, PRIMARY - erythroblastosis, hemolytic anemia, pyruvate kinase deficiency, sickle cell disease and variants, spherocytosis, thalassemia and variants

ANEURYSM - arteriosclerotic, arteriovenous (incl. fistula, malformation), dissecting, false, mycotic, poststenotic, syphilitic (See ANGIOMA)

ANGIOMA - hemangioma (incl. capillary, cavernous), angiographically occult vascular malformation

ARTERIOVENOUS MALFORMATION (AVM) - common vascular malformation with feeding arteries and draining veins

BLEEDING OR CLOTTING DISORDER - anticoagulant effect, coagulopathy (eg, disseminated intravascular type-DIC), hemophilia, purpura (eg, Henoch-Schönlein), thrombocytopenia

COLLAGEN DISEASE - dermatomyositis, lupus erythematosus (SLE), polyarteritis nodosa, scleroderma, mixed connective tissue disease (MCTD), CREST S. (calcinosis-Raynaud's- sclerodactyly-telangiectasia)

FAT EMBOLISM - incl. diffuse embolization of fatty bone marrow (after fracture), amniotic fluid, or oily contrast medium

FUNGUS DISEASE - actinomycosis, aspergillosis, blastomycosis, coccidiomycosis, cryptococcosis (torulosis), candidiasis (moniliasis), histoplasmosis, mucormycosis, nocardiosis

HAMARTOMA - a benign nodule composed of mature cells that normally occur in the affected part

HISTIOCYTOSIS X - eosinophilic granuloma, Hand-Schüller-Christian disease, Letterer-Siwe disease (nonlipid histiocytosis)

IMMUNOLOGIC DISORDERS - agammaglobulinemia (Bruton S.) or dysgammaglobulinemia, AIDS, ataxia-telangiectasia S., Bloom S., Buckley S., combined deficiency S., DiGeorge S., chronic granulomatous disease of childhood, Job S.

LYMPHOMA - includes Burkitt's lymphoma, Hodgkin's disease, non-Hodgkin's lymphoma, leukemia (all varieties, including chloroma), pseudolymphoma

---